# GASTRIC CARCINOGENESIS

# GASTRIC CARCINOGENESIS

Proceedings of the 6th Annual Symposium of the
European Organization for Cooperation in
Cancer Prevention Studies (ECP),
London, UK, 7–8 March 1988

*Editors:*

**Peter I. Reed**
Gastrointestinal Unit
Wexham Park Hospital
Slough, UK

**Michael J. Hill**
PHLS Centre for Applied Microbiology and Research
Bacterial Metabolism Research Laboratory
Salisbury, UK

 **1988**

**EXCERPTA MEDICA**, Amsterdam – New York – Oxford

International Congress Series No. 795
ISBN 0 444 81019 6

*Published by:*
Elsevier Science Publishers B.V.
(Biomedical Division)
P.O. Box 211
1000 AE Amsterdam
The Netherlands

*Sole distributors for the USA and Canada:*
Elsevier Science Publishing Company Inc.
52 Vanderbilt Avenue
New York, NY 10017
USA

*Library of Congress Cataloging in Publication Data*:

```
European Organization for Cooperation in Cancer Prevention Studies.
  Symposium (6th : 1988 : London, England)
    Gastric carcinogenesis : proceedings of the 6th Annual Symposium
of the European Organization for Cooperation in Cancer Prevention
Studies (ECP), London, UK, 7-8 March 1988 / editors, Peter I. Reed,
Michael J. Hill.
      p.   cm. -- (International congress series ; no. 795)
    Includes bibliographies and index.
    ISBN 0-444-81019-6 (U.S.)
    1. Stomach--Cancer--Congresses.  2. Stomach--Cancer--Etiology-
-Congresses.   I. Reed, P. I.   II. Hill, M. J.   III. Title.
IV. Series.
    [DNLM: 1. Stomach Neoplasms--etiology--congresses.  2. Stomach
Neoplasms--prevention & control--congresses.   W3 EX89 no. 795 / WI
320 E89g 1988]
  RC280.S8E87 1988
  616.99'433--dc19
  DNLM/DLC
  for Library of Congress                            88-24349
                                                        CIP
```

Printed in The Netherlands

# Foreword

ECP (European Organisation for Cooperation in Cancer Prevention Studies) was established in 1981 with the object of fostering the development of studies of aetiology and prevention of cancer on a European basis, since the activities of EORTC (European Organisation for Research on Treatment of Cancer) were restricted to research on cancer treatment.

Since then annual symposia have been devoted to themes of high priority for cancer prevention: "Tobacco and Cancer" (1983), "Hormones and Sexual Factors in Human Cancer Aetiology" (1984), "Diet and Human Carcinogenesis" (1985), "Concepts and Theories in Carcinogenesis" (1986) and "Causation and Prevention of Colorectal Cancer" (1987).

While sitting over a particularly good dinner in Budapest when attending the International Cancer Congress in August 1986 the editors conceived the idea of bringing together the leading experts in the field of gastric carcinogenesis in an attempt to shed more light on the aetiology and especially the prevention of a cancer which, while steadily decreasing over the past 30 years, is still numerically one of the most common cancers worldwide. We were particularly gratified by the fact that only one of the list of participants then drawn up could not attend the eventual meeting.

This volume contains the proceedings of the 1988 ECP symposium held in London, UK at the Royal College of Physicians, on March 7th and 8th on "Gastric Carcinogenesis". The aim was to review our current knowledge of this topic under four headings: "Background", "General Aetiology", "Gastric luminal factors" and "The Future". The high level of contributors ensured an outstanding overview of this clinical problem, highlighting the benefits which improvements in socio-economic factors have already achieved in the past three decades, but also stressing the need for further preventive measures to be agreed, including the initiation of intervention trials in high risk groups, to reduce further the incidence of this lethal disease. The symposium was enriched by an especially valuable poster session, the abstracts of which have been published in a special issue of "Cancer Letters" (Vol 39, Suppl. March 1988).

We are indebted to the speakers for their contribution during the symposium and for their prompt submission of manuscripts. We are grateful to the sponsors, Glaxo PLC and Miss Mandy Lakin of Gardner–Caldwell Associates for assistance with the smooth running of the meeting.

Our special thanks go to Mrs Belinda Johnston for all the work associated with the organisation of the meeting, Miss Theresa Gallagher for preparing and typing the camera ready forms of all the manuscripts and Dr Steve Leach, Craig Mackerness, Kathy McPherson and Philip Packer for their assistance in checking these afterwards.

We hope that this will be the first of a series of symposia on gastric carcinogenesis to be held in the future.

The 1989 ECP Symposium will be on "Aetiological and epidemiological relationships between cancers of the breast, endometrium and ovary" to be held in Bilthoven (The Netherlands) on 1–2 May 1989.

Peter I. Reed
Michael J. Hill

# Symposium speakers

Professor P. CORREA
Department of Pathology
Louisiana State University
Perdido Street
New Orleans LA 70112
USA

Professor M. CRESPI
Istituto Regina Elena
Viale Regina Elena 291
00161 Rome
Italy

Mr. F.T. DE DOMBAL
Clinical Information Science Unit
University of Leeds
22 Hyde Terrace
Leeds LS2 9LN
UK

Professor A.T. DIPLOCK
Division of Biochemistry
UMDS, University of London
Guy's Hospital
London Bridge
London SE1 9RT
UK

Professor J.B. ELDER
Academic Surgical Unit
Department of Postgraduate Medicine
University of Keele
Staffs ST4 7NK
UK

Dr. M.I. FILIPE
Department of Histopathology
UMDS, University of London
Guy's Hospital
London Bridge
London SE1 9RT
UK

Dr. S.P. GREEN
Division of Cancer and Control
National Cancer Institute
Bethesda MD 20892
USA

Dr. M.J. HILL
Division of Pathology
PHLS-CAMR
Porton Down
Salisbury, Wilts SP4 OJG
UK

Professor T. HIRAYAMA
Institute of Preventive Oncology
1-2 Ichgaya-Sadohara
Shinjuku-ku
Tokyo 162
Japan

Professor J.V. JOOSSENS
Department of Epidemiology
Universitaire Ziekenhuizen Sint-Rafael
Capucinijnenvoer 33
B-3000 Leuven
Belgium

Dr. P.A. JUDD
Department of Food and
Nutritional Sciences
Kings College London
Campden Hill Road
London W8 7AH
UK

Professor M.J.S. LANGMAN
Department of Medicine
Queen Elizabeth Hospital
Birmingham B15 2TH
UK

Mr. N.McC. MORTENSEN
John Radcliffe Hospital
Oxford OX3 9DU
UK

Dr. N. MUNOZ
Unit of Field and Intervention Studies
International Agency for Research
on Cancer
150 Cours Albert Thomas
69372 Lyon Cedex 08
France

Professor J. MYREN
Department of Gastroenterology
Ulleval University Hospital
Oslo 4
Norway

Dr. H. OHSHIMA
International Agency for Research
on Cancer
150 Cours Albert Thomas
69372 Lyon Cedex 8
France

Professor R. PREUSSMANN
Institute of Toxicology
German Cancer Research Center
P101949
D-6900 Heidelberg
FRG

Dr. B. RATHBONE
Department of Medicine
St James University Hospital
Leeds LS9 7TF
UK

Dr. P.I. REED
Department of Endoscopy
Wexham Park Hospital
Slough, Berks SL2 4HL
UK

Dr. C.L. WALTERS
Department of Biochemistry
University of Surrey
Guildford, Surrey
UK

Dr. C.E. WEST
Department of Human Nutrition
Wageningen Agricultural University
6703 BC Wageningen
The Netherlands

Dr. K.G. WORMSLEY
Ninewells Hospital
Ninewells, Dundee DD2 1UB
UK

# Contents

# BACKGROUND

© Elsevier Science Publishers B.V. (Biomedical Division)
Gastric carcinogenesis. P.I. Reed, M.J. Hill, editors.

# DIAGNOSIS AND SURGICAL TREATMENT OF GASTRIC CANCER

JAMES B ELDER
Academic Surgical Unit, Department of Postgraduate Medicine, University of Keele,
Thornburrow Drive, Hartshill, Stoke-on-Trent, UK

## INTRODUCTION

The diagnosis of gastric cancer at an early stage is often a very difficult feat. In countries where the disease has a very high incidence eg Japan (67 cases per 100,000 per annum), the application of mass screening or early diagnostic techniques can identify several cases at an early stage, as well as giving an initial high yield of some advanced cases on a large scale (26). In the United Kingdom the incidence of gastric cancer is much lower (27 cases per 100,000 per annum) and in common with most other countries in the world it has been declining steadily over the past 40 years. A recent survey (Fig. 1) defining the incidence in relation to age of the population in the United Kingdom reminds all of us involved in clinical work, to raise the index of suspicion of the diagnosis in patients over the age of 50 who have vague, persistant, yet often very mild upper gastrointestinal symptoms. From the data (Fig. 1) gastric cancer below the age of 25 is rare but in the fourth and fifth decades there is a steadily increasing incidence of the disease in both males and females. Another helpful strategy is the identification within the population of special high risk groups in which, for one reason or another, there appears to be an increased risk of the disease developing. A list of well-known groups at risk and risk factors is given in Table 1.

### Diagnosis

Many diverse factors can help us in arriving at the diagnosis of early gastric cancer, not least of which is the fact that in a recent UK survey (de Dombal, personal communication) about 50-60% of cases were, in fact, symptomatic. This has been emphasised by Allum and his colleagues in Birmingham (2), whose open-access endoscopy clinic for males with persistant dyspepsia lasting longer than 6 weeks resulted in a higher pick-up rate than previously achieved in that region of the UK, together with a higher percentage of cancers at an earlier and operable stage. It can be seen from Table 1 that many of the conditions and groups listed result from a suppression of normal gastric acid secretion with hypo-or achlorhydria often associated with damage to the epithelium. Some of the detailed factors operating at the mucosal level will be discussed elsewhere in this book.

4

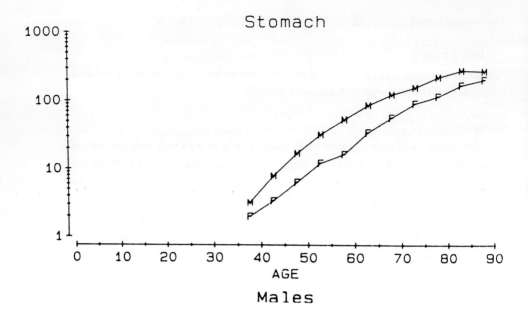

Fig. 1. Age-related incidence of gastric cancer in United Kingdom (Source: Registrar General Statistics).

TABLE 1

IDENTIFYING FACTORS AND GROUPS ASSOCIATED WITH INCREASED RISK OF DEVELOPMENT OF GASTRIC CANCER

Blood group A
Pernicious anaemia
Chronic atrophic gastritis
Intestinal metaplasia
Gastric resection
Bile reflux
Geographic and ethnic factors
Diet and salt intake
Truncal vagotomy

Team Approach

In order to efficiently achieve a diagnosis of early gastric cancer, it is essential that colleagues form diagnostic teams comprising of a clinician with a high index of suspicion of the disease, an endoscopist (who may be the clinician), a motivated radiologist and pathologist. It is particularly important that a pathologist experienced in the diagnosis of dysplasia and of early gastric cancer is available (14,13).

## Clinical Diagnosis

From the point of view of clinical diagnosis any areas of suspicion in the stomach should be biopsied particularly using the "spiked" forceps to obtain tissue below the mucosal surface, and if possible at least 10 biopsies within a circumscribed area should be obtained. Biopsy alone is not sufficient and brush cytology can also be extremely helpful in establishing the diagnosis but requires the availability of an experienced gastric cytologist. It is now widely accepted that fiberoptic endoscopy with biopsy and brush cytology forms the gold standard for the critical diagnosis of gastric carcinoma (3,38). Nevertheless, endoscopy has not been 100% successful in diagnosing cases particularly in areas of difficulty, for example at the oesophago-gastric junction. Mori et al (42) have shown that certain cases of early gastric cancer (EGC), a diagnosis made in 21 patients out of a total of 2,237 cases of gastric cancer, all lay within 2cms below the cardio-oesophageal junction and the lesions themselves varied from 1 to 4cms in size. The diagnostic point at issue lies in the fact that in 16 of their 21 cases of EGC of the cardia, the diagnosis was directed and suspicions raised by a double contrast barium meal study, so that the endoscopist could be guided to the particular area in question. This important clinical contribution also pointed out that these early gastric cancers in this part of the stomach were coincident in some cases with duodenal ulcer, gastric ulcer in others and, in a few cases, early gastric cancer was found elsewhere in the stomach. The role of radiology is also emphasised in a further recent pospective study of 385 patients with 'dyspepsia' by Shaw et al (1987) (58) who submitted their cases to double contrast barium meal and endoscopy without allowing either speciality access to the findings of the other. Analysis of the results in terms of diagnosis of gastric cancer suggested that carefully performed double contrast radiology of the stomach in some hands can compete with equal merit with that of fiberoptic endoscopy. In practice most patients will have an endoscopy and in cases of difficulty or doubt all diagnostic methods should be employed. Both diagnostic techniques are labour intensive of clinicians' time and have cost implications particularly relevant in countries where the incidence of the disease is relatively low, such that mounting large scale screening programmes, particularly by endoscopic methods, are beyond the means of available resource. This situation applies in the United Kingdom.

## Histological and Morphological Classification

Our Japanese colleagues have been pioneers in clarifying the endoscopic

6

classification of early gastric cancer which is now used as a standard by endoscopists the world over (Fig. 2). This classification based on simple luminal morphology of possible lesions has, moreover, allowed endoscopists to examine critically mucosal abnormalities and has helped in the precise location of the site selected for biopsy (35).

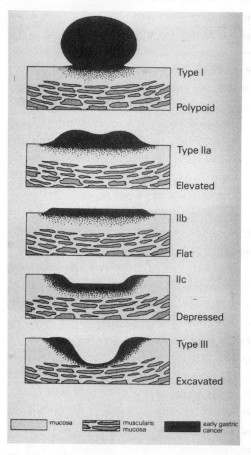

Fig. 2. The Japanese morphological classification of gastric cancer (Illustration reproduced by kind permission of Gower Medical Publishing Co).

A histological classification of gastric cancer from the work of Lauren (36) more than 20 years ago described two broad groups: the diffuse type and the intestinal type. Recent evidence has strongly suggested that the frequency of the diffuse type of carcinoma decreases markedly with increasing age, while the incidence of the intestinal type accounts for over 60% of cases at the age of 70 or more (24). Clinically the world-wide decline in gastric cancers has primarily been found in those suffering from the intestinal type, strongly suggesting that it is a change in environmental factors which may well be responsible for this decrease (60,27,44). As in all pathological classifications there is some degree of overlap with areas of both types being seen in the one specimen and in a minority of cases (<10%) classification on this system is not possible at all.

## Staging of Gastric Carcinoma - Relationship to Survival

A prime determinant of surgical treatment after making the diagnosis is the stage of the cancer. We are again indebted to our Japanese colleagues for defining the microscopic staging of early gastric cancer as adopted by the Japanese Cancer Research Society in 1963 (13). Early gastric cancer, therefore, has been defined as confined to the mucosa or submucosa as determined by depth of infiltration of the gastric wall, but has been associated with lymph node metastases in 15-20% of cases. The implication for successful surgical treatment is well-illustrated by the report of Takasugi et al (62) who showed that the post-operative 10-year actuarial survival rate for early gastric cancer confined to the mucosa was 100% and for that in the submucosa 95%.

## Is there a Change in Clinical Pattern?

Changes in the clinical pattern of gastric carcinoma in North America and in England have recently been noted (41,47) suggesting that proximally based tumours have increased in frequency whereas carcinomas of the antrum and body have significantly decreased in incidence over the past 30 years (p>0.01). Whether these simply reflect the better diagnostic facility offered by the fiberoptic endoscope, or are a true reflection of a change of location of the disease with time will require further study from other geographic locations, but if such reports are confirmed then a greater index of suspicion and greater vigilance in the area of the cardia and proximal stomach will be required.

## The Gastric Ulcer Dilemma

The diagnosis of gastric cancer associated with a gastric ulcer presents the clinician with difficulty. A recent report by Rolag and Jacobson (1984) (52) has helped to clarify these issues. 121 gastric ulcers benign at original assessment by biopsy and brush cytology were traced after 6 years. Many had undergone surgery for their original gastric ulcer on the dictum adopted by many clinicians that "if the ulcer fails to heal within 6 months, gastrectomy is advised because of the risk of malignancy". Others (n = 17) had died from unrelated causes and 22 with no clinical complaints who were traced refused further investigation, and 4 could not be found. However, a substantial majority (n = 78) were re-scoped and had multiple biopsies taken from the site of the previous ulcer or from any suspicious areas in the stomach. One gastric cancer was found. None of the original ulcers removed at surgery were found to be malignant. This report emphasises the safety with which predictions can be made if a gastric ulcer is thoroughly assessed at the initial endoscopy, sampled by biopsy and brush cytology and serves to remind us that most gastric cancers are not associated with a classic gastric ulcer (10).

Tumour Markers - Future Possibilities?

The search for suitable markers for gastric cancer has intrigued many workers in recent years, particularly with the availability of monoclonal antibodies to the neoantigens Ca19-9, Ca50, Ca12-5 as well as the existing spectrum of oncofetal antigens originating with CEA (23). The problem has been that while some cancers are clearly identified, most of the markers are not sensitive or specific enough to be used routinely in vivo for the detection of gastric carcinoma (48,34). Recent studies with murine monoclonal antibodies with restricted antigen epitopes on CEA are more hopeful, picking up 72% of a pilot series (45). Since the majority of gastric cancers are associated with a degree of gastritis an exciting possibility using the serum pepsinogen groups 1 and 2 both individually and as a ratio as described by Samloff et al (55) might allow us to define the histologial state of the gastric mucosa from a simple serum sample submitted to the respective radioimmunoassays (Fig. 3). If applied on a mass scale after validation from the original reports in the siblings of a Finnish cohort with pernicious anaemia, then such a strategy may allow the definition of high risk groups with atrophic gastritis and hyposecretion, who could then be further investigated by endoscopy and cytology. Unfortunately the antibodies and antigens are not yet widely available particularly for the group 2 pepsinogens (ie those associated with the antrum of the stomach).

Another exciting possibility not only for identification of patients with gastric cancer but of malignancy in many other locations could result from application of the techniques described by Fossel et al (15,16). This group made use of the magnetic resonance-water-suppressed proton spectrum associated with the methyl and methylene groups in the lipoproteins of plasma. They described the almost complete separation of patients with varying types of adenocarcinoma including those of the stomach and the colon from age and sex matched normal subjects, and from the majority of those hospital control patients suffering from non-cancer diseases. However, the details in this report do not in any way reflect the stage of the tumour.

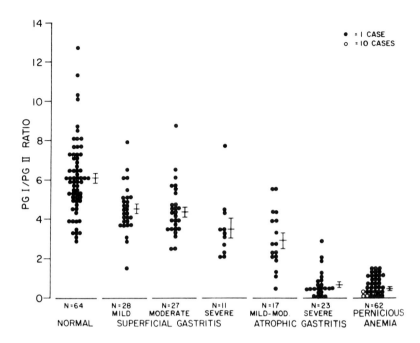

Fig. 3. The relationship between the ratio of Group I pepsinogens to Group II pepsinogens in the serum of siblings of pernicious anaemia cases and the histology of the stomach (by kind permission of Dr M Samloff, and Gastroenterology).

Gastric Polyps - A High Risk Group

Most polyps in the stomach are pseudoinflammatory and have nothing to do with gastric cancer (11) but the adenomatous polyp can undergo malignant change (Fig. 4). They are often seen incidentally in the investigation of a patient with mild dyspepsia or with gastrointestinal bleeding, and there is good prospect in the future that treatment by endoscopic laser techniques will allow ablation of such lesions without resort to gastrectomy (51).

Surveillance of the Post-Operative Stomach

Cancer of the gastric stump after gastrectomy or after truncal vagotomy and drainage for peptic ulcer has long been known by the relevance of the pre-operative diagnosis, the age of the patient at the time of original surgery, the particular

TABLE 2
CARCINOMA AFTER GASTRIC SURGERY - COHORT STUDIES

| Author | Reference | Country | Type | No | FU (%) | Comparison | Risk |
|--------|-----------|---------|------|-----|--------|------------|------|
| Krause 1957 | (33) | Sweden | Billroth II | 385 | 96 | I Rates | 2.2* |
| Helsingen et al | (22) | Norway | Gastrectomy | 229 | 76 | I Rates | 2.1* |
| Liavaag 1962 | (37) | Norway | Gastrectomy | 616 | 91 | I Rates | 1.0 |
| Hakkiluoto 1976 | (18) | Finland | Gastrectomy | 171 | 98 | I Rates | 0.4 |
| Domellof et al 1977 | (9) | Sweden | Gastrectomy | 534 | 78 | I Rates | 1.4 |
| Ellis et al 1979 | (12) | England | Gast or V&D | 1024 | 94 | % Rate | |
| Ross et al 1982 | (53) | Scotland | Gastrectomy | 856 | 91 | Mort Rate | 0.8 |
| Caygill et al 1986 | (6) | England | Gast or V&D | 5018 | 90 | I Rates | 3.7+ |
| Viste et al 1986 | (69) | Norway | Gastrecomy | 3470 | <100 | I Rates | 2.1+ |

* p < 0.01
+ p < 0.001
I Rates = Incidence rates in that country

operation performed, the definition of control populations for comparison and the necessary duration of follow-up in such cases have all been addressed in recent communications. Green (19), in an endoscopic survey of 163 patients at a median post-operative time of 14.6 years after gastric resection for benign ulcer disease found 3 resectable adenocarcinomas in the gastric stump. He concluded, controversially, that yearly screening by endoscopy should be performed after a 10 year post-resection interval, and re-emphasised the point that endoscopy and biopsy were preferable to upper gastrointestinal barium contrast studies where the anatomy is more difficult to interpret having been altered by surgery. Similar advice is given by Saario et al (54) regarding endoscopic follow-up of cases of "curative partial resection" for gastric cancer. Studies addressing the question of risk of development of gastric cancer after gastric surgery for benign conditions are grouped in Table 2 (cohort studies (33,22,37,18,9,12,53,6,65) and Table 3 (case control studies (61,31,46,56). It is clear that in some countries previous peptic ulcer surgery is undoubtedly associated with an increased risk of developing gastric cancer but not in others eg the USA where no significant increase in incidence of gastric cancer after gastrectomy or vagotomy has been consistently demonstrated. It may well be that local environmental factors are important as well as previous gastric surgery. Of particular interest is the report by Caygill et al (6) which differentiates clearly for the first time the risks following surgery for ulcer surgery was followed by a decreased risk of gastric cancer in the first 20 post-operative years, when the initial surgery had been a gastrectomy, whereas it increases in gastric ulcer patients. After truncal vagotomy and drainage for DU a susceptible part of the stomach namely the antrum remains and is associated with bile reflux and possible antral mucosal damage, possibly conferring an earlier risk of developing carcinoma than the situation after gastrectomy.

The question of the mechanisms involved in development of gastric cancer after vagotomy and drainage was elegantly addressed in a study by Watt and Kennedy of 144 patients originally undergoing either vagotomy and gastrojejunostomy (n=82) or vagotomy and pyloroplasty (n=62) and compared at 15-25 years after surgery with an age and sex matched healed duodenal ulcer population (67). All patients had endoscopy and several gastric biopsies. Moderate and severe dysplasia in the antrum were significantly increased in those after surgery and an increase in intestinal metaplasia was noted particularly after vagotomy and gastroenterostomy (p<0.01). No frank carcinoma of the stomach was found in this relatively small group who all had operations initially for benign disease. A sub-group of 33 patients in whom bilious vomiting was clinically a problem underwent bile diversion and were rebiopsied one year later. The incidence of dysplasia in mucosal biopsies was significantly decreased even after this short time of freedom from significant bile

TABLE 3
CARCINOMA AFTER GASTRIC SURGERY - CASE CONTROL STUDIES

| Author | Reference | Country | Type | No | Comparison | Risk |
|---|---|---|---|---|---|---|
| Stalsberg et al 1971 | (61) | Norway | Gastric Ca | 630 | Autopsy controls | 2.9* |
| Kivilaakso et al 1977 | (31) | Finland | Gastric Ca | 464 | Autopsy controls | 1.8 |
| Papachristou et al 1980 | (46) | USA | Gastric Ca | 1496 | GI cancer controls | 3.0* |
| Sandler et al 1984 | (56) | USA | Gastric Ca | 521 | Community control | NS+ |

reflux (p<0.002). A further detailed analysis of this question of the role of bile reflux is given elsewhere in this book by Mortensen (43).

## Surgical Treatment of Carcinoma of the Stomach

Successful surgical treatment of carcinoma of the stomach by resection employing partial or in appropriate cases total gastrectomy depends on the stage of the disease at the time of operation. It has been established by our Japanese colleagues that cases of early gastric cancer, ie where the tumour microscopically is confined to the mucosa or submucosa, even although as many as 15-20% will have lymph nodes involved, surgical treatment is followed by 90% five year survival (28,29,30). This experience is not limited to the Japanese population: reports of similar, excellent results have appeared from North America (17,5,20), Italy (50) and Canada (49). The frequency of early gastric cancer coming to surgical treatment in non-Japanese countries is well below 10% in most series in contrast to more than 40% detected by mass survey techniques in Japan (29).

## TNM Staging and Correlation with Operative Staging

Microscopic surgical staging of gastric carcinoma using 'the TNM system' (21) has been applied in a recent study, the aim of which was to establish the accuracy with which a surgeon could stage the disease clinically at operation (40). It is extremely important that each patient should have an operation appropriate to the stage of disease and Madden's report emphasises that good assessment at operaton is not a terribly accurate excercise, being correct for the tumour size and depth of penetration in 60% of cases and predicting involved lymph nodes in a similar percentage compared to histopathological examination of the specimens. Naturally, liver metastases were detected in 92%, but surgical curability assessed conservatively on the TNM system as $T_{1-3}, N_{0-1} M_0$ was correct only in 8 of 18 patients assessed. Incurability, perhaps easier to define, was pathologically correct in 58 of 60 patients. Despite inaccurate surgical staging no patient was denied a resection, although in this series of 78 consecutive operations for gastric cancer, 10 patients had unduly radical procedures for their stage. The position is well summarised in an accompanying leading article (8).

Improved methods of prediction of operability using endoscopic ultrasonography (EUS) are suggested by Hayder and Lux (25) who claim very accurate assessment of the depth of penetration of cancer particularly in the oesophagus and stomach but numbers studied are small. The concept of radical surgery removing all involved lymph nodes on first principles suggests that a better outcome will result and experience in Japan supports this, and a prospective randomised trial currently underway in the United Kingdom may provide scientific proof. The general message for surgeons is clear: we need to improve our methods of operative staging in order to offer appropriate surgery.

Extent of Gastric Resection

Controversy still reigns as to whether surgery for most gastric cancers means literally total removal of the stomach, the view of Schlag (57), or whether lesser procedures would be more appropriate. This latter view is supported by Lundell et al (39) who warn of the high complication rates associated with gastric cancer surgery especially when partial pancreatectomy is added to gastric resection. Of crucial importance in operable cases, however, whether it is partial or total resection, is clearance at the resection line. Analysis by the British Stomach Cancer Group (4) leaves little room for complacency. They documented cancer positive resection lines in 85 (22%) of 390 gastric cancer resections with the expected poor prognosis of survival. In 32 instances this occurred at the oesophageal resection margin, 20 at the proximal gastric margin, 17 at the duodenal margin with disease being left in the duodental stump and in 6 cases both proximal and distal levels had not been cleared. Since resection-line disease is apparently unfortunately all too common, intraoperative measures such as frozen section should theoretically allow control. However, complete sampling of resection lines with immediate pathological examination could be too time-consuming for many centres, in view of the large number of sections required and so clinical experience and surgical judgement are still the mainstay in the operative assessment and treatment.

Geographical Variation in Results of Surgery for Gastric Carcinoma

Results of surgical treatment of advanced gastric cancer can vary quite significantly within one country. The analysis by Silman (59) shows that within England 5 year survival rates vary from 3-4% in the north and east of the country to 11% in the Home counties and the London region where population density is greatest. No reasons are provided in this report but the differences suggest further study is warranted.

Sadly many patients do not seek medical advice at a time when the disease has produced very mild symptoms, and equally many practitioners discouraged by the results of surgery in advanced cases still all too often fail to refer cases in which there may be reasonable grounds for suspecting the diagnosis, on the basis that seldom in our current practice will it be possible to offer anything worthwhile. Such pessimism is not justified and requires a change of attitude and, at national level, the importance of provision of adequate and early endoscopic facilities for all in whom suspicion of the disease is raised must be recognised.

Is there a Need for Surgical Follow-up After Operations for Gastric Cancer?

The question of whether we should follow up our cases of gastric cancer after surgery outside a research endeavour or protocol is an important one and must be linked to the possibility of future clinical intervention with benefit. Two recent studies address this problem and provide useful data: firstly Viste et al (66) studied

206 cases of established or advanced cancer at the time of gastric resection. The five year survival of this series was 13%. 19 of 83 "curative resections" were found on follow-up to have recurrent carcinoma proven by biopsy and of those 10 came to laporotomy and all were found to be unresectable. This accords with a conventional clinical view that it is seldom possible to have surgical intervention after the initial resection for established gastric carcinoma. By contrast a study by Koga et al (32) of 452 cases of EGC followed for longer than 5 years identified 15 with gastric recurrence in which further surgical treatment was possible and, interestingly, 10 patients with carcinoma of other organs such as kidney, lung, breast and prostate. This report emphasises the need for follow-up after surgery for EGC and an awareness that this population may well have increased susceptibility to cancer at other sites.

## New Techniques in Assessment of Gastric Cancer

Yesuda et al (68) detected submucosal tumour of the order of 5mm in size using endoscopic ultrasound (EUS) in 83 patients but did not clearly define criteria for operability of lesions. An attempt at staging lesions in the oesophagus and stomach was made by Tio et al (63) using EUS: in 36 cases of gastric carcinoma EUS was accurate in defining resectability in 9 of 11 actually coming to surgery, and in forecasting palliative resection correctly in 13 out of 15 cases confirmed at operation, with non-resectability predicted in 8 out of 10 cases. These results are very encouraging but a note of caution is sounded by Aibe et al (65) who found that although enlargement of lymph nodes could be detected by EUS in gastric cancer, pathological examination of the large nodes did not always confirm that enlargement was due to metastatic cancer. Magnetic resonance may improve the situation but we await further detailed studies. Clearly computed tomograpahy (CAT scanning) has been disappointing in its ability to predict resectability in gastric cancer (64,7). Laparotomy and thorough intraoperative assessment are still at present required in cases of gastric or suspected gastric cancer in whom there is even a small chance of resectability. Surgical follow-up and check gastroscopy are mandatory after surgery for all cases of EGC for life.

## REFERENCES

1. Aibe T, Ito T, Yoshida T, Noguchi T, Ohtani T, Takemoto T (1986) Scand J Gastroenterol 21 (Suppl 123):164-169

2. Allum WH, Hallessey MT, Dorrell A, Low J, Fielding JWL (1986) Br Med J 293:541

3. Bringage WL, Chappuis CW, Cohn I, Correa P (1986) Ann Surg 204:103-107

4. British Stomach Cancer Group (1984) Br Med J 289:601-603

5. Carter KJ, Schaffer HA, Ritchie WP Jr (1984) Ann Surg 199:604-609

6. Caygill CPJ, Hill MJ, Kirkham JS, Northfield TC (1986) Lancet i:929-931

7. Cook AO, Levine BA, Sirinaulk KR, Gaskill HV (1986) Arch Surg 121:603-606

8. Cushieri A (1986) Br J Surg 73: 513-514

9. Domellof L, Eriksson S, Janunger KG (1977) Gastroenterology 73:462-468

10. Editorial (1985) Lancet i:202

11. Elder JB (1987) In: Misiewicz JJ, Pounder RE, Venables CW (eds) Diseases of the Gut and Pancreas, Blackwell Scientific Publications, Oxford pp371-380.

12. Ellis DJ, Kingston RD, Brookes VS, Waterhouse JAH (1979) Br J Surg 66:117-119

13. Fernando SSE, Nakamura K (1986) Am J Gastroenterol 81:757-763

14. Filipe MI, Potet F, Bogomoletz WV, Dawson PA, Fabiani B, Cheuveinc P, Fenzy A, Gazzard B, Goldfain D, Zeegen R (1985) Gut 26:1319-1326

15. Fossell ET, Car JM, McDonough J (1986) N Eng J Med 315:1369-76

16. Fossell ET, Carr JM, McDonough J (1987) N Eng J Med 316:1415

17. Gentsch HH, Groith H, Giedl J (1981) World J Surg 5:103-107

18. Hakkiluoto A (1976) Am Chir Gynaecol 65:361-368

19. Green FL (1987) Arch Surg 122:300-303

20. Green PHR, O'Toole KM, Weinberg LM et al (1981) Gastroenterology 81:247-256

21. Harmer MH (1978) 3rd edition UICC, Geneva 63-67

22. Helsingen N, Hillestad L (1956) Ann Surg 143:173-179

23. Heptner G, Domschke S, Domschke W (1986) Hepato-gastroenterol 33:140-144

24. Hermanek P (1986) Hepato-gastroenterol 33:180-183

25. Heyder N, Lux G (1986) Scand J Gastroenterol 21 (suppl 23):47-57

26. Hirayama T (1981) In: Fielding JWL et al (eds.) Gastric Cancer. Pergamon Press, Oxford, pp77-84

27. Hirayama T (1981) In: Fielding JWL, Newman CE, Ford CHJ, Jones BG (eds.) Gastric Cancer. Advances in Biosciences Vol 32, Pergamon Press, Oxford

28. Kabakino T, Nei H, Abe T et al (1975) Gastroenterol Jpn 10:1-5

29. Kaneko E, Nakamura T, Umeda N et al (1977) Gut 18:626-630

30. Kato K, Kito T, Nakazato H et al (1975) Nagoya J Med Sci 38:35-42

31. Kivilaakso E, Hakkiluoto A, Kalima TV, Sipponens P (1977) Br J Surg 64:336-338

32. Koga S, Kaibara N, Tamura H, Mishidoi H, Kimura O (1984) Surgery 96:511-516

33. Krause U (1957) Acta Chir Scand 114:341-354

34. Janssen CW, Maartmann-Moe H, Lie RT (1987) Europ J Oncol 13:285-295

35. Japanese Research Society for Gastric Cancer (1981) Jpn J Surg 11:127-139

36. Lauren P (1965) Acta Pathol Microbiol Scand 64:31-49

37. Liavaag K (1962) Ann Surg 155:103-106

38. Longho WE, Bucker KA, Zdon MJ, Ballantyne SH, Cambria RP, Modlin IM (1987) Arch Surg 122:292-295

39. Lundell L, Grip J, Olbe L (1986) Acta Chir Scand 152: 145-149

40. Madden MV, Price SK, Learmonth GM, Dent DM (1987) Br J Surg 74:119-121

41. Meyers WC, Damiano RJ, Postlethwait RW, Rotolo FS (1987) Ann Surg 205:1-80

42. Mori M, Kitagawn S, Iida M, Sakurai T, Enjoji M, Sugimachi K, Owiwa T (1987) Cancer 59:1758-1766

43. Mortensen NJMcC (1988) In: Reed PI, Hill MJ (eds) Gastric Carcinogenesis. Elsevier, Amsterdam pp

44. Munoz N (1988) Cancer Letters 39:Suppl 58

45. Ohuchi N, Wunderlich D, Fuyita J, Colcher D, Muraro R, Nose M, Schlom J (1987) Cancer Res 47:3565-3571

46. Papachristou DN, Agnanti N, Fortner JG (1980) Am J Surg 139:193-198

47. Paterson IM, Easton DF, Corbishley CM, Gazet JC (1987) Br J Surg 74:481-482

48. Quentmeier A, Schlag P, Geisen HP, Schmidt-Gayk H (1987) Europ J Surg Oncol 13:197-201

49. Rheault MJ, Leandri R, Lapointe A et al (1981) Can J Surg 24:606-607

50. Ribichini A, Piccinini E, Perucci A et al (1984) Int Surg 69:325-329

51. Rickey GD, Descon JA (1981) Gastrointest Endoscopy 27:224-225

52. Rollag A, Jacobson CD (1984) Acta Med Scand 216:105-109

53. Ross AHM, Smith MA, Anderson JR, Small WP (1982) N Eng J Med 307:519-522

54. Saario I, Schroder J, Lempenion M, Kiwilaakso E, Nordling S (1987) Arch Surg 122:1052-1054

55. Samloff IM, Varis K, Ihamaki T, Siurala M, Rotter JI (1982) Gastroenterology 83: 204-209

56. Sandler RS, Johnson MD, Holland KL (1984) Dig Dis Sci 29:703-708

57. Schlag P (1986) Europ J Surg Oncol 12:235-2395

58. Shaw PC, van Romunde LKJ, Griffoen G, Janssens AR, Kreuning J, Eilep GAM (1987) Radiology 163:39-42

59. Silman AJ (1985) Hospital Update 11:735-745

60. Silverberg E (1986) Cancer Statistics CA 36:9-25

61. Stalsberg H, Yaksdal S (1971) Lancet ii:1175-1177

62. Takasugi T, Hirota T, Sasagowa M (1977) Stomach Intestine 12:993

63. Tio TL, Den Hartog Jager FCA, Tytgat SNJ (1986) Scand J Gastroenterol 21 (Suppl 123):71-86

64. Triller J, Roder R, Stafford A, Schroder R (1986) Europ J Radiol 6:181-186

65. Viste A, Bjonestad E, Opheim P, Skarstein A, Thonold J, Hartveit F, Eide GE, Eide TJ (1986) Lancet ii:502-505

66. Viste A, Rygh AB, Soreide O (1984) Clin Oncol 10:325-332

67. Watt PCH, Sloan JM, Spencer A, Kennedy TL (1983) Br Med J 287:1410-1412

68. Yasuda K, Makajima M, Kawai K (1986) Scand J Gastroenterol 21 (suppl 123) 59-67

© Elsevier Science Publishers B.V. (Biomedical Division)
Gastric carcinogenesis. P.I. Reed, M.J. Hill, editors.

# INTESTINAL METAPLASIA IN THE HISTOGENESIS OF GASTRIC CARCINOMA

M ISABEL FILIPE

Department of Histopathology, UMDS, Guy's Hospital, London SE1 9RT, UK

## INTRODUCTION

Despite the decreasing incidence of gastric carcinoma worldwide, it still remains an important health problem in Western Europe and many parts of the world but, unlike other cancers, cure is possible. Detection of gastric carcinoma at an early stage (EGCa) offers an excellent prognosis with 5-year survival rates, after surgery, at 97.6% and 91.8% for the intramucosal and submucosal EGCa respectively (17).

Fundamental to the screening of populations to select those at higher risk of gastric cancer, is a knowledge of early events and their better definition. The majority of gastric carcinoma, particularly the 'intestinal' type (Lauren's classification) (13) develop in a background of intestinal metaplasia, and there is strong evidence for the chronic atrophic gastritis -- , intestinal metaplasia -- , dysplasia -- , carcinoma sequence, concept proposed by Correa (5) and some of these aspects will be referred to by Professor Correa in this monograph (3).

Dysplasia is a well recognised premalignant change. In practice, however, a screening protocol based solely on the presence of dysplasia in gastric biopsies has its limitations due to the focal nature of the lesion, the uncertainty regarding the histological criteria, its low incidence (2-3%) in the endoscopic biopsies, and the fact that its presence often co-exists with established carcinoma (2,20). On the other hand, intestinal metaplasia is a common lesion (20-30% of gastric biopsies), easy to define and its incidence is higher in high risk as compared to low risk gastric cancer areas (4). However, its presence in both benign and malignant conditions has limited its potential use as indicator of cancer risk.

We will focus on intestinal metaplasia and attempt to discuss the following aspects:

## HETEROGENEITY OF INTESTINAL METAPLASIA

The heterogeneity of intestinal metaplasia (IM) has been recognised by ultrastructure (19), enzymatic profile (28), mucin secretion (12), and antigenic expression (6,18) and various classifications have been proposed (7,9,22,26,30). Based on morphology and mucin secretion, three main IM phenotypes have been identified (7):

Type I (also termed "mature", "complete", or "small intestinal" type): regular architecture and straight crypts lined by mature absorptive and goblet cells. Goblet cells secrete sialomucins and occasionally neutral and/or sulphomucins. Absorptive cells are non-secretory and present a brush border. Paneth cells are often seen (Figure 1).

20

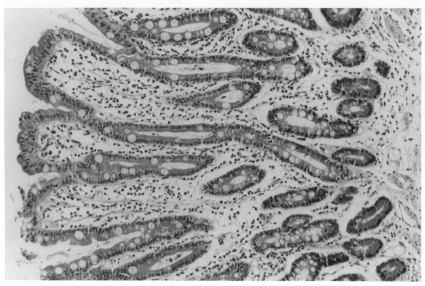

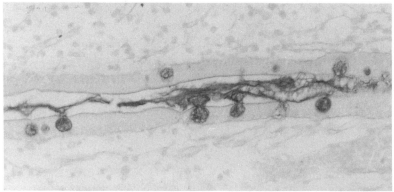

Fig. 1. Intestinal metaplasia type I: upper- straight crypts lined by mature absorptive and goblet cells. H & E stain. lower- On HID/AB stain absorptive cells are non-secreting and goblet cells secrete sialomucins (grey). H & E x 64; HID/AB x 160.

Type II (incomplete): mild architectural distortion, elongated and slightly tortuous crypts lined by goblet cells, fewer mature absorptive cells and increasing numbers of columnar cells with apical mucus secretion. These contain neutral and/or sialomucin. The goblet cells secrete sialo- and occasionally sulphomucins. Paneth cells are rare or absent.

Type III (immature "incomplete" or "colonic" type): variable degree of architectural distortion and tortuosity of crypts, with marked cellular dedifferentiation. Columnar cells secrete predominantly sulphomucins and goblet cells contain sialo- and/or sulphomucin. Paneth cells are inconspicuous (Figure 2).

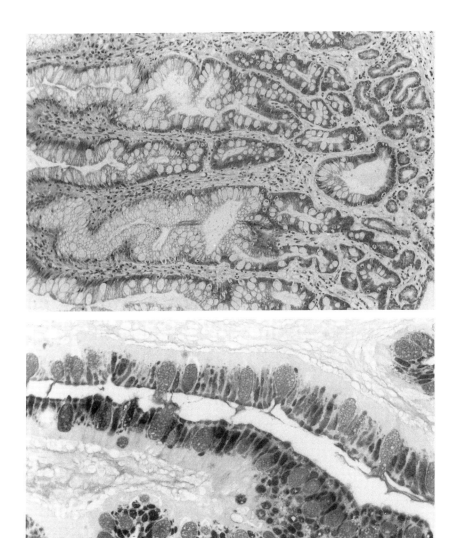

Fig. 2. Intestinal metaplasia (incomplete) type III: (a) The crypts are tortuous and lined by columnar mucous cells and interspersed goblet cells. (b) On HID /AB columnar cells secrete predominantly sulphomucins (black) and goblet cells contain a mixture of sialo-(grey) and/or sulphomucins (dark grey/black). H & E x 64; HID/AB x 160.

Sulphomucin in goblet cells can be detected in any IM type and its significance is not known. Similarly, the presence of sulphomucins in sites not showing IM, such as the base of antral and pyloric glands, within cysts and in mucus neck cells. Forms of transition between these three categories are observed and often co-exist in an individual case.

Other variants of intestinal metaplasia, have been described, based on the staining patterns of goblet cells mucous secretion, particularly its content in O-acylated sialomucins (22).

Despite different classifications of IM and terminology used, there has been general agreement that sulphomucin positive incomplete = colonic, = type III variants are significantly associated with gastric carcinoma of intestinal type, whilst type I and II are not.

INTESTINAL METAPLASIA PHENOTYPES AND GASTRIC DISEASE

Our data on gastric biopsies, collected from four different centres, show 20-30% incidence of intestinal metaplasia, which is prevalent in gastric carcinoma (65%) (8,23). Type I IM is the most common (approximately 70%) and the prevalent type in all conditions. The non-sulphated incomplete type shows an even prevalence (20-25%) in chronic gastritis, gastric ulcer and carcinoma. In contrast, type III IM was found in approximately 10% of the IM positive biopsies. This represents only 5% of IM positive biopsies in chronic gastritis and gastric ulcer, compared with 36% in carcinoma. It thus seems that the non-sulphated phenotypes I and II are common to both benign conditions (approximately 95%) and carcinoma (64%), and that type III is more selective for carcinoma (Figure 3). Similar results have been described by others (21,25), and its high prevalence (77-80%) in mucosa adjacent to EGCa and microcarcinomas has been well documented in gastrectomy specimens by Japanese authors (11,16). It is important to note that intestinal metaplasia is more common in the "intestinal" than in the "diffuse" type of gastric carcinoma, and the values for type III IM, in gastrectomy specimens, in our series are 67% and 9% for IGCa and DGCa respectively (23).

INTESTINAL METAPLASIA PHENOTYPES
Incidence and Distribution in Gastric Biopsies
(n = 2391)

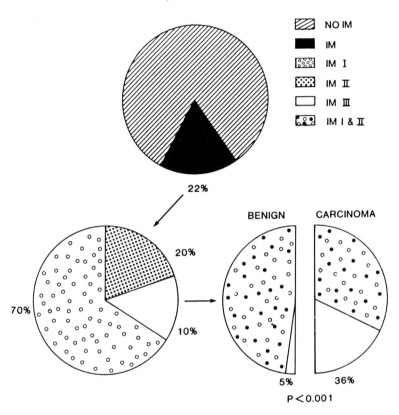

Fig. 3. Intestinal metaplasia phenotypes: Incidence and distribution in gastric biopsies (n = 2391).

INTESTINAL METAPLASIA IN THE EVOLUTION OF CHRONIC GASTRITIS AND GASTRIC ULCER: ITS RELATIONSHIP WITH SEVERITY OF INFLAMMATION AND HEALING

(a) Preliminary data on 216 biopsies from a 5 year prospective follow-up study of 58 patients with chronic gastritis and intestinal metaplasia in the initial biopsy, seem to indicate that the inflammatory background differs in Types I and III IM. Type I appear to be related to the severity and activity of the gastritis, whereas type III was more often seen in the absence of significant inflammatory infiltrate and this pattern remained unchanged during the follow-up period. Furthermore, 30 of the 47 patients with initial type I IM, reverted to normal. In contrast, of the 8 patients with initial type III IM, the same feature persisted during follow-up, associated with dysplasia in 5 of these patients and carcinoma developed in one of them, 4 years after the initial biopsy (24).

(b) Similarly, preliminary data on 227 biopsies from a 5 year prospective follow-up study of 67 patients with gastric ulcer and intestinal metaplasia in the initial biopsy, suggest a relationship between type I IM and disease activity, whilst type III IM appeared to be independent of its course, being more common in cases of delayed ulcer healing and reactivation (24).

The significance of these changes, particularly the presence of intestinal metaplasia with abnormal mucin phenotypes, is not yet known, but may have a marked effect on the functional gel forming properties of mucus, which have been shown to occur in peptic ulcer. These changes in mucin composition may lead to a weaker gel structure, hence a poor protective cover to the mucosa in those patients (1).

## CAN WE DISCRIMINATE BETWEEN REACTIVE AND PRE-NEOPLASTIC PHENOTYPES OF INTESTINAL METAPLASIA?

The concept that types of intestinal metaplasia with different morphological and mucin profiles may have a different risk of gastric malignancy, has support from early reports on intestinal marker enzymes, and recent studies on antigenic expression, proliferative activity and DNA analysis (Table 1).

TABLE 1

INTESTINAL METAPLASIA PHENOTYPES

|  | Carcinoma vs Non-Carcinoma patients | | References |
|---|---|---|---|
| Sulphomucins: |  |  |  |
| Biopsy | 36% | 5% | Filipe et al (8) |
| Gastrectomy | 77% | 14% | Silvia & Filipe (23) |
|  |  |  | Hirota et al (11) |
| Antigens: |  |  |  |
| LIMA | + | - | Filipe et al (6) |
| $M_3C$ | + | - | Nardelli et al (18) |
| Proliferative activity (LI) | 35.8% | 13% | Steenback & Wolff (27) |

Depending on enzyme markers of small intestinal differentiation, intestinal metaplasia has been classified into "complete" and "incomplete" (28). Complete IM shows the enzyme profile of small intestine with sucrase, trehalase, aminopeptidase (AMP) and alkaline phosphatase (ALP). In incomplete IM, various enzymes are reduced or absent and these include ALP, trehalase, and to a lesser extend AMP. Incomplete IM has been shown to be prevalent in intestinal gastric carcinoma (77-80%) (11,16).

Mucus-associated antigens, prepared form extracts of foetal and adult intestinal mucosa and carcinoma, have been used to elucidate cell lineage and cell differentiation in gastrointestinal carcinogenesis (6,10,18). The expression of large intestinal mucin antigen (LIMA) has been demonstrated in the gastric epithelium of carcinoma-bearing stomachs (29/30, 97%) but not in benign controls. The antigenic expression correlates well with dysplasia (100%) and type III IM (100%). Of particular interest, however, is the detection of abnormal cell populations expressing the antigen within type I IM (60%) and type II IM (85%), in the carcinoma group, but not in the controls (6) (Table 2).

TABLE 2

LARGE INTESTINAL MUCIN ANTIGEN (LIMA) IN STOMACH RESECTED FOR CARCINOMA

| Histology | LIMA+/Total | % |
|-----------|-------------|------|
| Normal | 0/30 | 0 |
| IM I | 13/22 | 59% |
| IM II | 17/20 | 85% |
| IM III | 18/18 | 100% |
| Dysplasia | 20/20 | 100% |
| Carcinoma | 19/30 | 63% |
| Patients | 29/30 | 97% |

Key: IM = Intestinal metaplasia
     I,II, and III= Types

Similarly, other intestinal mucin antigens expressed in goblet cells of normal adult small intestine ($M_3SI$), duodenal villi ($M_3D$) and large intestine ($M_3C$) also appear to discriminate between intestinal metaplasia in benign conditions, which reveal $M_3SI$ and $M_3D$ and IM adjacent to carcinoma which expresses $M_3C$ (in addition to $M_3D$ and $M^3SI$ antigens) (18) (Table 1).

The phenotypes described in intestinal metaplasia within carcinoma fields, as opposed to controls, are shared by the majority of gastric carcinomas particularly the intestinal type, and in some aspects resemble foetal gut (10,18).

Furthermore, the labelling index of intestinal metaplasia in patients with gastric cancer has been reported as 3-fold higher than in non-cancer patients (14) (Table 1). To probe this concept, studies designed to correlate proliferative activity, abnormal phenotypes and patterns of DNA synthesis are needed (15,29,31).

CLINICAL IMPLICATIONS OF THE PRESENCE OF INTESTINAL METAPLASIA IN GASTRIC BIOPSIES

We have illustrated an association between certain variants of IM and intestinal type gastric carcinoma but their precancerous nature has not yet been established in long term follow-up studies on a large series of subjects.

We consider that incomplete IM III satisfies the criteria for mild dysplasia: cellular atypia, abnormal differentiation and distorted mucosal architecture, and in view of the available data it should be regarded as a risk factor in terms of patient follow-up, and one of the parameters to be included in any screening programme for gastric cancer. At present, guidelines for follow-up surveillance cannot be given with any measure of precision.

Two studies are now in progress which attempt to answer some of these questions in a relatively short-term:

1. A retrospective study using large number of patients, whose records for periods of 10-20 years were available, and previous gastric biopsies used for mucin typing of intestinal metaplaisa. The aim is to obtain data on the natural history of IM in general and type III IM in particular.*

2. The ECP-Euronut Intestinal Metaplasia study is a prospective study involving 2,000 subjects from various European countries. The histological criteria for test patients is the presence of intestinal metaplasia including mucin typing of IM. A protocol for endoscopy and histology designed by a panel of pathologists and gastroenterologists in this group can provide a guideline for similar studies in other centres (see Appendix)**.

* IARC study

** European Organisation for corporation in cancer prevention studies. Workshop held in Wageningen, 5-7th May 1986

REFERENCES

1.   Allen A, Garner A, Keogh JP (1986) In: Filipe MI, Jass JR (eds) Gastric Carcinoma. Churchill Livingstone, Edinburgh, pp256-273

2.   Camilleri JP, Potet F, Amat C, Molas G (1984) In: Ming SC (ed) Precursors of Gastric Cancer. Praeger Publ. New York, pp83-92

3.   Correa P (1988) Precancerous lesions of the stomach. In: Reed PI, Hill MJ (eds) Gastric Carcinogenesis. Elsevier, Amsterdam pp

4.   Correa P, Cuello C, Duque E (1970) J Natl Cancer Instit 44:297-306

5.   Cuello C, Correa P (1979) In: Herpath CL, Schlag P (eds) Gastric Cancer. Springer-Verlag, Heidelberg, pp83-90

6.   Filipe MI, Barbatis C, Sandey A, Ma J (1988) Human Pathol 19:19-26

7.   Filipe MI, Jass JR (1986) In: Filipe MI, Jass JR (eds) Gastric Carcinoma. Churchill Livingstone, Edinburgh, pp87-115

8.   Filipe MI, Potet F, Bogomoletz WV et al (1985) Gut 26:1319-1326

9.   Heilmann KL, Hopker WW (1979) Pathol Res and Practice 164:249-258

10.  Higgins PJ, Correa P, Cuello C, Lipkin M (1984) Oncology 41:73-76

11.  Hirota T, Okada T, Itabashi M et al (1984) In: Ming SC (ed) Precursors of Gastric Cancer. Praeger Publ, New York, pp179-193

12.  Jass JR, Filipe MI (1979) Histopathology 3:191-199

13.  Lauren P (1965) Acta Pathol Microbiol Scand 64:31-49

14.  Lehnert T, Deschner EE (1986) In: Filipe MI, Jass JR (eds) Gastric Carcinoma. Churchill Livingstone, Edinburgh pp45-67

15.  Lipkin M, Correa P, Mikol IB et al (1985) J Natl Cancer Inst 75:613-619

16.  Matsukura N, Zuzuki K, Kawachi T et al (1980) J Natl Cancer Inst 65:231-240

17.  Nagayo T (1986) Histogenesis and precursors of human gastric cancer. Research and Practice. Springer-Verlag, Heidelberg

18.  Nardelli J, Bara J, Rosa B, Burtin P (1983) J Histochem Cytochem 31:366-375

19.  Nevalainen TJ (1986) In: Filipe MI, Jass JR (eds) Gastric Carcinoma. Churchill Livingstone, Edinburgh, pp236-255

20.  Oehlert W (1979) In: Herpath CL, Schlag P (eds) Gastric Cancer. Springer-Verlag, Berlin, pp91-104

21.  Rothery GA, Day DW (1985) J Clin Pathol 38:613-621

22.  Sugura DI, Montero C (1983) Cancer 52:498-503

23.  Silva S, Filipe MI (1986) Human Pathol 17:988-995

24.  Silva S, Filipe MI, Pinho A (1988) (in preparation)

25.  Shipponen P (1981) Ann Clin Res 13:139-143

26.  Shipponen P, Seppala K, Varis E et al (1980) Acta Pathol Microbiol Scand 88:217-224

27.  Steenbeck L, Wolff G (1971) Arch Gescwulstforsch 38:132-8

28.  Sugimura T, Kawachi T, Kogure K et al (1973) In: Nakahara W et al (eds) Differentiation and Control of Malignancy of Tumour cells. University of Tokyo Press, pp251-261

29.  Szentirmay Z, Csuka O, Sugar J (1986) In: Filipe MI, Jass JR (eds) Gastric Carcinoma. Churchill Livingstone, Edinburgh, pp68-85

30.  Teglbjaerg PS, Nielsen HO (1978)  Acta Pathol et Microbiol Scand 86:351-355

31.  Teodori L, Capurso L, Cordelli E et al (1984) Cytometry 5:63-70

© Elsevier Science Publishers B.V. (Biomedical Division)
Gastric carcinogenesis. P.I. Reed, M.J. Hill, editors.

# WHAT FACTOR IS RESPONSIBLE FOR MALIGNANT CHANGE IN THE RAT STOMACH FOLLOWING TRUNCAL VAGOTOMY AND GASTROENTEROSTOMY?

P R TAYLOR, D C HANLEY, M I FILIPE AND R C MASON
Departments of Surgery and Histopathology, UMDS (University of London), Guy's Hospital, London SE1 9RT, UK

This study was designed to investigate the role of truncal vagotomy and duodenogastric reflux (DGR) resulting from gastroenterostomy in gastric carcinogenesis in the rat. Male Wistar rats (250g) received either a gastrotomy-controls or a gastroenterostomy -GE or a truncal vagotomy and gastroenterostomy-TVGE. After 9 months they were sacrificed and samples obtained for intragastric pH measurement and histological assessment of high grade dysplasia and carcinoma. The results are shown below.

|          | No of Rats | pH (mean + LSD) | No with Dysplasia/Carcinoma |
|----------|------------|-----------------|------------------------------|
| Controls | 11         | 3.9 + 2.1       | 0                            |
| GE       | 12         | 3.7 + 2.7       | 8 (68%)                      |
| TVGE     | 12         | 7.3 + 1.2       | 3 (25%)                      |

Intragastric pH was significantly higher in animals with TVGE when compared to controls (t=4.7,p<0.001), and GE (t=4.2,p<0.001). No difference was found between controls and GE. High grade dysplasia and carcinoma occurred more often in GE animals than controls (Chi$^2$=8.5,p<0.01) but no significant difference was detected between TVGE and GE nor between controls and TVGE.

No evidence was found to implicate vagotomy in the malignant process but these results confirm that DGR is an important factor in gastric carcinogenesis in the operated rat stomach. As this role does not appear to be pH related, DGR probably exerts its effect directly on the gastric mucosa rather than via overgrowth with nitrate reducing bacteia.

© *Elsevier Science Publishers B.V. (Biomedical Division)*
*Gastric carcinogenesis. P.I. Reed, M.J. Hill, editors.*                                              31

$I^{125}$-EGF RADIO RECEPTOR BINDING STUDIES IN NORMAL HUMAN GUT
EPITHELIAL CELL MEMBRANES, ANTRAL CARCINOMA AND COLONIC
ADENOCARCINOMA

S A CARTLIDGE AND J B ELDER
Academic Surgical Unit, Department of Postgraduate Medicine, University of Keele,
Stoke-on-Trent, UK

Membrane preparation from 30 specimens comprising normal gut mucosa, antral
gastric carcinoma and carcinoma of the colon were made after removing the tissues
at surgery and snap freezing them in liquid nitrogen. The mucosa was separated
from the muscle layer after thawing. Using $I^{125}$ iodine labelled EGF, specific
binding was of the order of 10-58% of the labelled peptide exposed to a membrane
preparation obtained from the tissues (Table).

| Tissue Type | N | Amount EGF Bound (pm/mg protein) $\pm$ SD | $K_D$ (M) | Non-specific Binding |
|---|---|---|---|---|
| Normal asc. colon | 4 | 0.03 $\pm$ 0.006 | 2.5 x $10^{-9}$ | 65 |
| Asc. colon carcinoma | 5 | 0.017 $\pm$ 0.002 | 7.9 x $10^{-10}$ | 42 |
| Normal desc. colon | 3 | 0.12 $\pm$ 0.04 | 4.5 x $10^{-10}$ | 71 |
| Desc. colon carcinoma | 2 | 0.09 | 8.0 x $10^{-10}$ | 63 |
| Normal sigmoid colon | 2 | 0.29 | 5 x $10^{-9}$ | 62 |
| Sigmoid carcinoma | 5 | 0.11 | 1 x $10^{-10}$ | 70 |
| Normal antrum | 3 | 0.05 $\pm$ 0.007 | 4.6 x $10^{-9}$ | 55 |
| Antral carcinoma | 3 | 0.03 $\pm$ 0.006 | 9 x $10^{-10}$ | 47 |
| Terminal ileum | 3 | 0.01 $\pm$ 0.005 | not obtainable | 90 |

Membranes from the epithelial cells from cancers of the stomach and colon
bound less than normal tissues but there was considerable variation. Such findings
may be due to the presence of endogenous and/or autocrine growth factors such as
TGF alpha occupying the EGF receptor. Preliminary results with fresh normal gut
mucosa obtained from a young adult kidney donor confirm different degrees of
binding of $I^{125}$-EGF in different areas of the gut, and acid washing at pH 4.5 after
exposure of the mucosal strips to the radio-labelled ligand followed by re-incubation
with fresh $I^{125}$-EGF resulted in increased binding, suggesting occupation of the EGF
receptors by endogenous peptides in the freshly obtained tissue. These studies have
important implications for the study of normal and cancerous epithelial cell
membranes containing the EGF receptor obtained freshly for binding studies.

© Elsevier Science Publishers B.V. (Biomedical Division)
Gastric carcinogenesis. P.I. Reed, M.J. Hill, editors.

# BRITISH SURVEY OF DYSPLASIA AND EARLY GASTRIC CANCER

F T DE DOMBAL

Clinical Information Science Unit, University of Leeds, 22 Hyde Terrace, Leeds LS2 9LN, UK

## INTRODUCTION

The dilemma faced by clinicians who deal with gastric cancer both in the UK and elsewhere, is well established and well recognised. As the cancer progresses, there is a rise in detectability - until once the "classical cancer syndrome" has developed, the proportion of cancers which can be readily diagnosed is very high. Unfortunately, at the same time the curability level falls - so that once the classical cancer syndrome has fully developed, the chance of cure by any modality treatment is small.

Moreover, high technology - efficient in itself - has not changed the situation much. In the 1950's diagnostic technology was primitive, the miss rate for gastric cancer in the UK was around 35% and the 5 year survival rate only 7%. Nowadays, with double contrast radiology, endoscopy, brush cytology and biopsy all readily available the miss rate is well under 10% - but unfortunately the 5 year survival rate has not changed much, and in many international studies is still under 10%.

## METHODS OF EARLIER DIAGNOSIS

Several means have been suggested by which this dismal situation can be improved. Whole population screening has been advocated in some quarters - though in the present impecunious state of the National Health Service it is highly unlikely that adequate facilities would be available in the UK for this remedy. Improvements in high technology are constantly suggested; but as already pointed out, high technology is currently very effective and any further improvements could only marginally effect the present situation. Concentration upon high risk groups has also many advocates. However, whilst this is inherently sensible, such high risk groups account for less than 10% of the current load of gastric cancers in the UK and elsewhere.

Reducing the "Lead-Time"

One disquieting feature of the present situation is the long "lead-time" between the development of symptoms and the establishment of a diagnosis of gastric cancer. MacAdam (4) demonstrated that this amounted to a median of six months - equally spread between delay in General Practice and delay in Hospital - between first consultation and the establishment of the diagnosis. It would be greatly advantageous if this lead-time could be reduced by alerting doctors to the features of early gastric cancer as opposed to the classical cancer syndrome. However, a major problem with this potential solution lies in the fact that the symptoms of early gastric cancer are almost totally unrecorded. Descriptions in the textbooks outline the "classical cancer syndrome" which (as already discussed) is of only marginal relevance in improving cure rates.

Herein lies the rationale into the study carried out by the British Society of Gastroenterology in order to identify a cohort of patients with early gastric cancer, and study their mode of presentation and clinical features. The results will now be described.

## THE BRITISH SOCIETY OF GASTROENTEROLOGY SURVEY

This survey was begun in the early 1980's and at present (1987/8) comprises a total of 319 patients. In all some 47 hospitals have contributed material via a total of 70 members of the British Society. The survey is on-going and the present discussion refers to an interim analysis of the first 126 cases.

### Quality Control

What is special about yet another investigation of early gastric cancer? It could cogently be argued that the B.S.G. survey, even when complete, might not contribute very much. The number of cases is small, and the survey can make no claim to represent early gastric cancer in the UK - merely early gastric cancer as seen by members of the British Society in an unselected and non-consecutive series of cases.

Nevertheless, it can also be argued that the B.S.G. survey has something valid to contribute - for reasons of quality control. Each case, from each centre, has been registered into the survey via a carefully constructed proforma designed to elicit specifics of clinical presentation. Moreover, pathological material from each case has been reviewed by a "panel" of three experienced pathologists and the "survey diagnosis" only arrived at after a strict review of the pathological material by the panel.

The effects of this area are considerable. Of the 126 cases referred into the survey, only a total of 66 were eventually categorised by the panel as "early gastric cancer" and another 16 as "dysplasia". No less than 29 cases were considered by the panel to have "advanced gastric cancer", 16 as "dysplasia", and 15 cases to have a miscellany of other conditions.

These results must give rise to some disquiet, not in relation to the B.S.G. survey, but in relation to other surveys. For if this degree of discrepancy extends between individual pathologists, it is difficult to place much credence upon surveys where the same form of quality control has not been instituted.

Presentation

The survey first enquired amongst the cases of early gastric cancer as to the mode of presentation, the chief symptom which brought the patient to the attention of the doctor in the first place. Overwhelmingly this was pain, 87% of the cases presenting with pain mostly in the epigastrium. Most of the remaining cases presented with upper GI bleeding. Between them these two modes of presentation accounted for all but a handful of cases (including one or two where the cancer seems to have been found as an incidental feature).

Clinical Features

Table 1 delineates the clinical features of these cases. 60% were male and 40% female, with a mean age of 63.1 years. Most patient's pain resembled that of peptic ulceration, being moderate in four-fifths of cases, and in half the patients being aggravated by food and/or relieved by antacids. Just under half of patients complained of nausea and one-third of vomiting. Loss of appetite and weight being present in about two-fifths.

TABLE 1

PRESENTATION OF EARLY GASTRIC CANCER

---

Clinical Features of 66 cases

| | | |
|---|---|---|
| * | 60% Male, | 40% Female |
| * | Man Age 63.1 years | range (40-80+) |
| * | Pain severity moderate 80% | |
| * | Aggravated by food | 48% |
| | Relieved by antacids | 43% |
| | Relieved by Cimetidine | 14% |
| * | Relation symptoms to meals | 64% |
| * | Nausea | 44% |
| * | Vomiting | 33% |
| * | Loss of appetite | 44% |
| * | Loss of weight | 46% |
| * | Previous surgery | 40%** |
| * | On $H_2$ Blockers | 32% |

---

** 3 cases DU surgery in distant past

Similarly two-fifths of patients had undergone previous surgery; but on closer enquiry the "classical" operative situation (peptic ulcer surgery in the distant past) was only present in three cases of those studied. Interestingly around half of patients had received $H_2$ blockers for a period of at least several months at the time their cancer was detected and most of these patients were still receiving this form of treatment at that time.

Endoscopy Features

The endoscopy features which were available in 47 cases are listed in Table 2. Even though interim these data provide some interest. For example, it is often alleged that the vast majority of patients in whom early gastric cancer is detected in the UK have their cancer detected in an otherwise benign chronic gastric ulcer. This was only the case in half of the current set of patients.

TABLE 2

PRESENTATION OF EARLY GASTRIC CANCER

Endoscopy findings in 47 cases

| Appearances: | Erosions | 3 cases |
|---|---|---|
| | Ulcers | 24 cases |
| | Other | 20 cases |
| Site: | Cardia | 2 cases |
| | Lesser curve | 25 cases |
| | Antrum/Pylorus | 15 cases |
| | Other | 5 cases |

COMPARISON WITH OTHER DISEASES

These data, interesting in themselves, require to be placed in context. Comparison between the principal symptoms in this series of early gastric cancer cases and similar series of cases with advanced gastric cancer, peptic ulcer and "functional" or non-ulcer dyspepsia are illustrated in Table 3. As shown, the symptoms of early gastric cancer more closely resemble peptic ulceration than they resemble either non-ulcer dyspepsia or advanced gastric cancer. The data in Table 3 reinforce the conclusion that there is an urgent need fr radical revision of the textbooks and clinical teachings if future medical students and clinicians are to be trained to identify early gastric cancer (as opposed to the classical cancer syndrome).

TABLE 3

COMPARISON WITH OTHER DISEASE CATEGORIES

Symptoms of early gastric cancer patients vs those patients with peptic ulcer (PU), functinal (FUNCT) and advanced gastric cancer (AGC) (2)

| No. of Patients | FUNCT | PU | EGC | AGC |
|---|---|---|---|---|
| | 100 | 100 | 100 | 100 |
| Epigastric Pain | 52% | 76% | 80% | 54% |
| Aggravated by Food | 16% | 26% | 48% | 8% |
| Related to Meals | 33% | 46% | 64% | 48% |
| Antacid Relief | 26% | 37% | 43% | 9% |
| Loss Appetite | 36% | 46% | 44% | 90% |
| Loss Weight | 32% | 55% | 46% | 85% |

COMPUTER ANALYSIS

Is it possible in some way to combine these features in order to obtain a prediction which will allow patients to be scheduled according to their risk of cancer and thereby brought to definitive investigation more quickly? Table 4, data from a study in Airedale, England, suggests that this might be the case. Most cancer cases in this series were scheduled by computer prediction into a "high risk" group to be investigated urgently by means of endoscopy. Such an arrangement (if practiced) might improve the hit rate of endoscopy and reduce thereby the lead-time between presentation and diagnosis (1). Moreover, these results have been repeated as far afield as N.W. China (3). It could be argued that these cases are late cancer cases; but analysis of the current British Society of Gastroenterology series indicates that the vast majority of early gastric cancer cases in this series were also placed by the same means firmly in the "high risk" category.

International Variation

Finally, it may be helpful to place these findings in context as regards other countries. Table 5 compares a well documented Japanese series with the findings from the present UK series. As illustrated, there is considerable difference between the two series in terms of the proportion of patients with epigastric pain, nausea, vomiting and particularly loss of appetite and weight loss. This may be due to earlier diagnosis in Japan, but equally it may be due to differences in categorization, or even to real differences between the two countries concerned.

TABLE 4

SCHEDULING ACCORDING TO RISK

Comparison of computer predicted risk group in final diagnosis in 1,000 cases of dysplasia (Davenport et al (1))

| Final diagnosis | Risk Category | | |
|---|---|---|---|
| | Low | Medium | High |
| Normal or minimal disease | 89% | 63% | 69% |
| Peptic ulcer | 10% | 36% | 19% |
| Cancer | 0.3% | 0.5% | 10% |
| Total cases | 301 | 432 | 308 |

TABLE 5

INTERNATIONAL COMPARISON

Comparison between UK series and Japanese series

| No of Cases | Japan (181) | UK (66) |
|---|---|---|
| Epigastric Pain | 54% | 80% |
| Aggravated by Food | 8.8% | 48% |
| Nausea/Vomiting | 23.2% | 44% |
| Loss Appetite | 14.3% | 44% |
| Loss Weight | 6.6% | 46% |

DISCUSSION

This latter point in the present context of this symposium is highly relevant. In other areas of clinical practice (such as inflammatory bowel disease) studies carried out by the World Organisation of Gastroenterology (5) with careful quality control have been able to shed considerable light on the difficult problem of international variation. Mindful of Asimov's dictum - that the problems of the world are of such magnitude that it is quite beyond the resources of any one nation to overcome them - there would seem to be an unanswerable case for international co-operation in this area, with stringent quality control, in an attempt to bring the same benefits in terms of early gastric cancer as have been seen in other areas of gastroenterology. If this symposium provides the necessary stimulus for such a survey, then in the view of the present author it will prove to have been well worthwhile.

## ACKNOWLEDGEMENTS

It is a pleasure to acknowledge the many colleagues without whom this study would not have been undertaken. First, the data processing staff for their skillful and meticulous analysis of the data; work which was supported by a grant from Pilkington Medical Systems Ltd - support which is acknowledged with gratitude. Second, the panel of pathologists; whose laborious but necessary studies have contributed enormously to the present survey. Finally and particularly, gratitude is expressed to the many clinical colleagues who have participated in this survey by forwarding material.

## REFERENCES

1. Davenport PM, Morgan AG, Darnborough A, de Dombal FT (1985) Brit Med J 290:217-220

2. Horrocks JC, de Dombal FT (1978) Gut 19;1:19-26

3. Li Zeng-lie, Hu Fu-le (1982) Chinese Med J 95(4):2933-296

4. MacAdam DB (1979) J R Coll Gen Pract 29:723-729

5. Myren J, Bouchier IAD, Watkinson G, de Dombal FT (1979) Scand J Gastroent 14;Suppl 56:1-27

© Elsevier Science Publishers B.V. (Biomedical Division)
Gastric carcinogenesis. P.I. Reed, M.J. Hill, editors.

OVERVIEW OF EARLY GASTRIC CANCER AND RESULTS OF AN ITALIAN SURVEY

MASSIMO CRESPI AND ANTONIO GRASSI
Istituto Nazionale Tumori "Regina Elena" World Health Organization Collaborating Centre for Stomach Cancer, 00161 Rome, Italy

INTRODUCTION AND OVERVIEW

The "early" stage of gastric cancer is defined as a cancer limited to the mucosa or to the mucosa and submucosa, regardless of the presence of regional lymph node metastases. It has to be considered as simply an initial step in the natural history of gastric cancer. The main reason for the interest of clinicians in such an entity are the outstanding results obtained in the long-term survival after surgery, now available from followup studies of up to 20 years. Early gastric cancer (EGC) limited to the mucosa shows a 20 years actual survival of 99.1%; when mucosal invasion is present, the figure is 90.2; the overall result is 95% (13). Outside of Japan the survival rates at 5 and 10 years are lower but are still encouraging (Table 1).

TABLE 1

ACTURIAL SURVIVAL IN NON JAPANESE CASE SERIES OF E.G.C.

| Authors | 5 Years | 10 Years |
|---|---|---|
| Houghton (1985) | 92% | 85% |
| Klimenkov (1984) | 83.2% | – |
| Guagbi (1982) | 93.3% | – |
| Saubier (1982) | 80.9% | 70% |
| Rheault (1981) | 95.3% | |
| Schmidt (1981) | 89% | |

The depth of parietal invasion is the key feature for the characterization of EGC and so a correct final diagnosis may only be obtained by serial histological sections of the entire surgical specimen. Since 1962 the classification of EGC accepted worldwide is the one issued by the Japanese Society of Gastroenterological Endoscopy (28), which is based on the endoscopic macroscopic appearance. The disagreement among the two concepts is only apparent: in fact we know today that endoscopy and x-rays may provide a diagnosis of EGC which is only suggestive, because it needs the final histopathological confirmation.

The basic problem in clinical practice is, therefore, to reach the diagnosis of stomach cancer in its "early" stage, and this is a goal which is not easy to fulfill. In fact, up to now, a really significant rate of EGC amongst the total diagnosis of stomach cancer has been obtained only in Japan. A percentage of 25.6 is reported even in general hospitals, whilst in many screening programmes an astonishingly high rate up to 57.9% has been obtained (Table 2). The time trend shows a continuous rise in the prevalence of EGC from 217 in 1962 to 2,400 in 1980 (9); in resected cases from the screening programme in Miyagi prefecture (14) the rate of early to total gastric cancer, which was 16% in 1960, reached with regular increases 66.5% in 1982.

TABLE 2

PERCENTAGE OF EGC IN ALL CASES OF SURGICALLY TREATED GASTRIC CANCER (JAPAN 1984)

| Author* | % EGC | Source of Cases |
|---------|-------|-----------------|
| Hirota (1984) | 46.6 | Cancer Institute |
| Hisamichi (1984) | 57.9 | Occupational Group Screening |
| Arisue (1984) | 45.2 | Mass Screening |
| Hisamichi (1984) | 45.3 | Mass Screening |
| Terada (1984) | 44.5 | Mass Screening |
| Okajima (1984) | 25.6 | General Hospitals |

Please contact authors for details of references.

These figures are the result of a nationwide effort towards screening and early detection based on widespread use of double contrast x-rays and fibreoptic endoscopy. The reduction of gastric cancer mortality in Japan is substantially due to early diagnosis and its consequences, as estimated by an analysis (25) which showed that of the factors involved in the decrease, 16% was related to screening and early diagnosis, 30.1% was due to the greatly improved long term survival of EGC cases and the residual 53.9% was the result of the reduction in incidence of gastric cancer.

In Europe the situation is radically different because gastric cancer has been steadily decreasing for the last 30 years and mortality rates are less than half those observed in Japan. No mass screening programmes have therefore been implemented and the relative rates of early to total gastric cancer are consequently lower. A multinational enquiry, performed in 1977 (20), showed a rate of early to total gastric cancer of 6.2%, in a total 39,953 gastric cancers detected in 244 centres in 21 countries. Since then other reports from individual centres in Europe, USA and Latin America have shown rates of early to total gastric cancers ranging from 4.6% to 16% (Table 3) (3,5,7,8,10,15,19,22,26). In Italy a detection programme performed in four oncological centres (from 1977 to 1980) (1) reported rates of early to total gastric cancer ranging from 7.1 to 16.2% (Table 4).

TABLE 3

PERCENTAGE OF EARLY GASTRIC CANCER AMONG GASTRIC CANCERS IN SELECTED STUDIES

| Author* | Year | % Early Gastric Cancer |
|---|---|---|
| Eitner K (Germany) | 1981 | 14 |
| Green PR (New York) | 1981 | 13.1 |
| Jirasek V (Prague) | 1981 | 7.0 |
| Schmidt E (Goppingen) | 1981 | 12.1 |
| Bergmann W (Berlin) | 1981 | 9.4 |
| Mennicken C (Mannheim) | 1984 | 16 |
| Italian survey | 1986 | 8.2 |
| Espejo H (Spain) | 1986 | 8.1 |
| Oleagoitia JM (Spain) | 1986 | 14 |
| Bringaze WL (New Orleans) | 1986 | 4.6 |

*Please contact authors for details of references

TABLE 4

PERCENTAGE EGC OF ALL CASES OF GASTRIC CANCER IN FOUR AREAS IN ITALY (ASTE, REF 1)

| Medical Centres | Total No Gastroscopies | % EGC of Total Gastric Cancers |
|---|---|---|
| Florence ('77-'80) | 1387 | 16.2 |
| Forli' ('74-'80) | 5103 | 7.1 |
| Genova ('77-"0) | 1875 | 10.1 |
| Rome ('78-'80) | 911 | 9.1 |

To gather more information on the prevalence of EGC in Italy we promoted in

TABLE 5
SURVEY OF EARLY GASTRIC CANCER IN ITALY (1986)

| | 1980 | 1981 | 1982 | 1983 | 1984 | 1985 | Total |
|---|---|---|---|---|---|---|---|
| No Gastroscopies (OGD) | 46,250 | 53,668 | 70,493 | 71,680 | 809,555 | 99,821 | 422,467 |
| No Gastric Cancer x 1.000 OGD | 34.0 | 32.3 | 32.0 | 26.9 | 26.6 | 20.3 | 11.670 |
| No EGC x 1.000 OGD | 2.2 | 2.2 | 2.2 | 2.3 | 2.0 | 2.6 | 955 |
| Percent EGC of Total Gastric Cancers | 6.0 | 6.4 | 6.4 | 7.8 | 7.1 | 11.2 | 8.2 |

1986 a nationwide enquiry (herewith reported) in the framework of the activities of the World Health Organization Collaborating Centre for Stomach Cancer which is based in our Institute.

## MATERIALS AND METHODS

A precoded standardized questionnaire was sent to the members of the Italian Society of Digestive Endoscopy (SIED) and of the Italian Association of Hospital Gastroenterological Centres where g.i. endoscopy is performed. In the SIED surgeons from general hospitals performing g.i. endoscopy are included in addition to the gastroenterologists and surgeons working in University Institutes. The questionnaire requested basic information on: (a) the number of gastroscopies performed yearly from 1980 to 1985; (b) the total number of gastric cancers and EGC found per year; (c) the total number of surgico-pathologically confirmed EGC; (d) the macroscopic type and localization of EGC

The total number of questionnaires sent was 1047. The final evaluation was based only on the cases of EGC with post-surgical histological confirmation. The regional distribution of the replies (northern, central and southern Italy) was also calculated.

## RESULTS

Of the 77 questionnaires returned, 66 were sufficiently complete for data analysis. It is important to underline that in Italy the majority of endoscopic and surgical interventions are performed in public institutions and that the doctors on the mailing list are the staff members of these institutions. Therefore each questionnaire brought the data of the centre and this explains the apparent large discrepancy between the total number of questionnaires sent and returned. The geographic distribution of the 66 centres which returned the questionnaires was 28 from northern, 20 from central, and 8 from southern Italy. The total number of gastroscopies reviewed from 1980 to 1985 (Table 5) was 422,467 and 11,670 cases of gastric cancer were detected. There was a steady increase in the rate of early to advanced gastric cancer, from 6% in 1980 to 11.2% in 1985, but a decrease in the number of gastric cancers detected per 1,000 endoscopies.

## DISCUSSION

As shown in our data, the total number of gastroscopies doubled in the 66 centres between 1980 and 1985, a clear demonstration of the increased awareness in Italy of the potentialities of endoscopy. A further demonstration of this is the relative decrease in the number of gastric cancers detected per 1,000 gastroscopies which was related not only to the decrease in the incidence of stomach cancer but to the more widespread use of endoscopy. In contrast, in the same period there was a real increase in the number of EGC detected, and also in the rate of early to total gastric cancer.

The uneven regional distribution of centres performing endoscopy and of endoscopic awareness between northern, central and southern Italy is also clearly evident from the data recording the mean annual increase in EGC and total gastric cancers, which demonstrated that in the south most of gastric cancers are still diagnosed in an advanced stage. It is also evident that great differences in the detection rate of EGC exist between Italy and Japan, (Table 2) where the proportion of EGC ranged from 25.6% to 57.9%, compared with the overall rate of 8.2% in our survey. This latter figure is quite similar to the one (6.2%) reported in a multicentre European enquiry (6). If we consider recent case series from individual centres in Italy, they provide higher figures than the national average (Table 6), the mean values of the rate calculated in the last 5 to 10 years ranging from 6.7% to 17.8% (2,4,6,11,23,24). The time trends, showing an increase of the proportion of EGCs reaching 28% are of notable interest. The comparison (Table 7) of the distribution of macroscopic types of EGC between our data and those from Japan and Europe (12,20) is also of interest. The various subtypes in our survey are similar to those found in the European one, but entirely different from the ones reported in Japan. Great differences exist between Japan and Italy, especially in the proportion of the depressed type of EGC (69.8 versus 26.6) and the proportion of the excavated type (5.5 versus 32.9). Possible explanations of this may include the different classification criteria and/or a genuinely different pattern of EGC subtypes in the two areas.

TABLE 6

PERCENTAGE EARLY GASTRIC CANCER OF TOTAL GASTRIC CANCERS IN SELECTED ITALIAN STUDIES

| Author | Year | EGC/GC (*) |
|--------|------|------------|
| Bearzi F | 1977-1983 | 13.1 |
| Biasco G | 1976-1982 | 15.3 |
| Candidi A | 1973-1981 | 17.8 |
| Grigioni WF | 1974-1981 | 14.4 |
| Pennelli N | 1980-1983 | 9.5 |
| Ravaioli A | 1971-1984 | 6.7 |

(*) = Early Gastric Cancer/Gastric Cancer

TABLE 7

MACROSCOPIC TYPES OF E.G.C. IN DIFFERENT COUNTRIES

|  | Japan (Hirota 1984) | Europe (Miller 1977) | Italy (1986) |
|---|---|---|---|
| Elevated (I, IIa) | 21,7 | 31.2 | 28.2 |
| Flat (IIb) | 3 | 10.5 | 12.3 |
| Depressed (IIc) | 69.8 | 30.5 | 26.6 |
| Excavated (III) | 5.5 | 27.1 | 32.9 |

Regardless of the macroscopic type and dimensions of the EGC, the crucial feature for long-term survival was always the depth of infiltration into the lamina propria, which may trigger the lymphatic spread (18) as shown in an analysis of different case series (Table 8), in which the percent of lymph node metastases is three times higher when the submucosa is involved. In the initial overview we have already shown how this factor affected the long term survival.

All the data shown point out the high efficacy in EGC of surgical treatment in EGC and which remains the treatment of choice. Local endoscopic laser treatment, although attempted in limited series of selected (mostly inoperable) cases (16,17,21,27), is still of debatable value. In fact, the rate of success falls from 67% to 25% when the submucosa is involved; eligible lesions are mostly the protruding ones, provided that the treatment is extended to the 5 cm of surrounding healthy mucosa and a precise staging is reached also employing ultrasound endoscopy.

In conclusion we may say that the persistent downward trend of gastric cancer in Italy is gives a false justification for a lower priority in allocating public health resources. In fact, stomach cancer is still one of the leading causes of death from malignancies in many regions, and is still a highly lethal neoplasia because of the late diagnosis of most of the cases. Even if population-based screening is hardly justified and poorly accepted, we would like to stress the importance of focussing the attention on early diagnosis, which appears to be beneficial from the data of selected centres in Italy and abroad. The expanded use of endoscopy must be considered the more appropriate means to deal with this problem together with a more widespread use of double contrast x-rays, as shown by the Japanese experience.

TABLE 8

FREQUENCY OF LYMPH NODE METASTASES AND DEPTH OF INVASION OF
E.G.C. (LEHNERT, REF 18, MODIFIED)

| Author* | Depth of Tumor Infiltration | | | |
| | Mucosa | | Sub Mucosa | |
| | No of patients | % of Patients with Metastases | No of Patients | % of Patients with Metastases |
| --- | --- | --- | --- | --- |
| Hirayama (1984) | 710 | 5.2 | 804 | 14.8 |
| Georgii (1982) | 108 | 1.9 | 114 | 12.3 |
| Meyer (1981) | 51 | 1.9 | 39 | 25.6 |
| Sowa (1981) | 88 | 0 | 174 | 13.2 |
| Grigioni (1980) | 22 | 0 | 24 | 16.7 |
| Kidokoro (1980) | 184 | 5.4 | 183 | 18.6 |
| Muhe (1980) | 47 | 6.5 | 49 | 8.0 |
| Murakami (1979) | 69 | 2.9 | 57 | 15.9 |
| Elster (1978) | 199 | 1.5 | 101 | 4.0 |
| Takagi (1976) | 129 | 8.5 | 140 | 20.7 |
| Niwa (1972) | 198 | 5.1 | 196 | 22.4 |

*Please contact authors for details of references

REFERENCES

1. Aste H, Amadori D, Maltoni C, Crespi M, Pugliese V, Pacini F, Casale V (1981) Acta Endoscopica 11:123-132

2. Bearzi I, Randaldi R (1986) In: "Carcinoma gastrico e lesioni precancerose dello stomaco" - Edited by Rugge M, Arslan - Pagnini C, Di Cario F, Edizioni Unicopli, Milano, 47-60

3. Bergemann W, Hener C, Niedobitek F, Dumke K, Hewkel K, Reichard H (1981) Exerpta Med Int Congr Ser 555:249-256

4. Biasco G, Paganelli GH, Azzaroni D, Grigioni WF, Merighi SM, Stioja R, Villanacci V, Rusticali AG, Lo Cuoco D (1987) Dig Dis Sci 32:113-120

5. Bringanze WL, Chappuis CW, Correa P, Cohn J Jr (1986) Ann Surg 204:103-107

6. Candidi Thommasi A, Lomi M, Soldi A, Guarducci AM, Calabrese E, Albertacci A (1985) Giornale Italiano End Dig 8:23-29

7. Eitner K, Bosseckert H, Koppe P, Fritze C, Kuhne-Heid R, Machnik G (1985) Dtsch 2. Vendan Stoffwechselkr 45:141-148

8. Espejo H, Navarrete J, Ayala L, Velasquez H (1986) Dig Dis Sci New Series 31:101s

9. Fukutomi H, Sakita T (1984) Jpn J Clin Oncol 14:169-179

10. Green PHR, O'Toole M, Keinbergl M, Goldfarb JP (1981) Gastroenterology

1:247-255

11. Grigioni WF, Bondi A, D'Errico A, Milani R, Villanacci V, Mancini AM et al (1986) In: "Carcinoma gastrico e lesioni precancerose dello stomaco". Edited by rugge M, Arslan - Pagnini C, Di Mario F, Edizioni Unicopli, Milano, pp93-114

12. Hirota T, Itabashi M, Daibo M, Kitaoka M, Oguro Y, Yamada T, Ichikawa H (1984) Jpn J clin Oncol 14:181-199

13. Ichikawa H, Yamada T (1985) In: Edited by Miller B (ed) "Screening     for cancer", Academic Press, London,  pp193-214

14. Isamichi S, Sugawara N (1984) Jpn J Clin Oncol 14:211-223

15. Jirasek V, Duorakova H, Setka J, Balas V, Jrasek A, Drazna E (1981) Ces K Gastroenterol 35:365-374

16. Kasugai T, Sugiura H, Iro Y, Kano T (1984) Nippon rinsho 42:2282-6

17. Kato H, Konaka C, Kowate N, Anishimiya K, Saito M, Kinoshita K, Saki H, Okitsu H, Kawaguchi M, Aizawa K (1985) Intrnitst (Berlin) 26:675-687

18. Lehnert T, Erlandson RA, Decosse JJ (1965) Gastroenterology 89:939-950

19. Mennicken C, Bohrer MH, Jung M, Manegold BC (1986) Dtsch Med Wochenschr 111: 255-258

20. Miller G, Froelichr P (1978) Z Gastroenterol 16:678-683

21. Oguro Y, Hirashima T, Tajiki H, Yoshida S, Yamaguchi H, Yoshimori M, Itabashi M, Ahirota T (1984) Jpn J clin Oncol 14:271-282

22. Oleagoitia JM, Echevarria A, Sandidrian JI, Ulacia MA, Hernandez-Calvo J (1986) Br J Surg 73:804-806

23. Pennelli N, Cecchetto A, Montaguti A, Danieli D, Portesan O, de Bernardin M (1986) In: Rugge M, Arsaln - Pagnini C, Di Mario F (eds) "Carcinoma gastrico e lesioni precancerose dello stomaco", Edizioni Unicopli, Milano, pp93-114

24. Ravaioli A, Ridolfi R, Liverani M (1985) Acta Endoscopica 15:299-306

25. Sasaki J, Akai S (1985) GANN 76:149-153

26. Schmid E, Gehl H, Braich E, Haag S, Lorentz H, Kovarik P (1981) Z Gastroenterol 19:51-55

27. Sugimura H, Kano T, fujiwara N, Kasugai T (1984) In: Okabe   H,   Honda   T, Oshiba S (eds) "Endoscopic Surgery", Elsevier, Amsterdam,  pp137-144

28. Tasaka T (1962) Gastroenterological Endoscopy 4:4

# DESCRIPTIVE EPIDEMIOLOGY OF STOMACH CANCER

NUBIA MUNOZ

Unit of Field and Intervention Studies, International Agency for Research on Cancer, 150 Cours Albert-Thomas, 69372 Lyon Cedex 08, France

## INTRODUCTION

Although the rates of stomach cancer are declining in most populations, in 1980 it still remained the most common cancer in both sexes on a worldwode basis (26). However, because of its continuing decline and the increasing trends in lung cancer, it probably today takes second place in the world after lung cancer. The magnitude of the problem varies with degree of development; in developing countries this cancer ranks second after cervical cancer while in developed countries it ranks fourth after lung, colorectal and breast cancer. Large differences in incidence among populations, and a continuous decline over the last four decades in most populations, are the outstanding epidemiological characteristics of gastric cancer, which suggest a predominant role for external environmental factors. However, despite a profusion of aetiological hypotheses, the main determinants for the geographical and temporal patterns of stomach cancer are still largely unknown. In this chapter, I will review the geographical distribution of stomach cancer in the world, using the most recent information available, as well as its urban/rural distribution, time trends and changes in the incidence in migrant populations. These epidemiological features will also be reviewed for the two main histological types of gastric cancer, intestinal and diffuse.

### Worldwide Occurrence

The worldwide occurrence of stomach cancer is reasonably well reflected in the mortality rates, since this cancer is generally fatal. Figures 1 and 2 give the age-standardized death rates for males and females during the period 1981-1986 for those countries included in the 1987 World Health Statistics Annual (34). The high rates for Japan, Chile, Dominica, Poland, Portugal and Singapore and the low rates for the United States and most European countries are the most noteworthy features. The mortality data given on a national basis can be supplemented by incidence figures from national and sub-national cancer registries. Table 1 gives the age-standardized and cumulative rates of stomach cancer for selected populations from "Cancer Incidence in Five Continents, Vol V" (19), and Table 2 shows the age-standardized incidence rates and age standardized gastric cancer ratios for selected populations from "Cancr Occurrence in Developing Countries" (25). Concerning the data from the latter publication, it should be kept in mind that the quality of the data varies widely among the different registries, that the rates given for a certain

*Males,* 1981–1986

## AGE–STANDARDIZED DEATH RATES FOR STOMACH CANCER

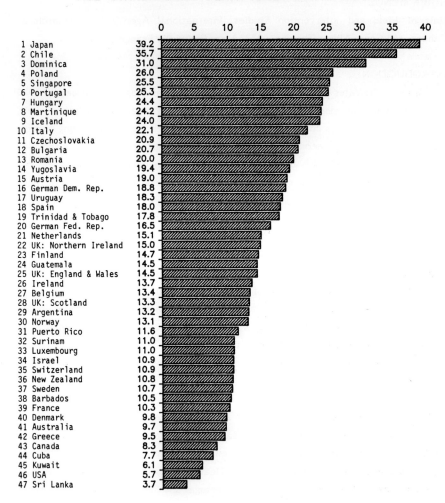

|  |  |  |
|---|---|---|
| 1 | Japan | 39.2 |
| 2 | Chile | 35.7 |
| 3 | Dominica | 31.0 |
| 4 | Poland | 26.0 |
| 5 | Singapore | 25.5 |
| 6 | Portugal | 25.3 |
| 7 | Hungary | 24.4 |
| 8 | Martinique | 24.2 |
| 9 | Iceland | 24.0 |
| 10 | Italy | 22.1 |
| 11 | Czechoslovakia | 20.9 |
| 12 | Bulgaria | 20.7 |
| 13 | Romania | 20.0 |
| 14 | Yugoslavia | 19.4 |
| 15 | Austria | 19.0 |
| 16 | German Dem. Rep. | 18.8 |
| 17 | Uruguay | 18.3 |
| 18 | Spain | 18.0 |
| 19 | Trinidad & Tobago | 17.8 |
| 20 | German Fed. Rep. | 16.5 |
| 21 | Netherlands | 15.1 |
| 22 | UK: Northern Ireland | 15.0 |
| 23 | Finland | 14.7 |
| 24 | Guatemala | 14.5 |
| 25 | UK: England & Wales | 14.5 |
| 26 | Ireland | 13.7 |
| 27 | Belgium | 13.4 |
| 28 | UK: Scotland | 13.3 |
| 29 | Argentina | 13.2 |
| 30 | Norway | 13.1 |
| 31 | Puerto Rico | 11.6 |
| 32 | Surinam | 11.0 |
| 33 | Luxembourg | 11.0 |
| 34 | Israel | 10.9 |
| 35 | Switzerland | 10.9 |
| 36 | New Zealand | 10.8 |
| 37 | Sweden | 10.7 |
| 38 | Barbados | 10.5 |
| 39 | France | 10.3 |
| 40 | Denmark | 9.8 |
| 41 | Australia | 9.7 |
| 42 | Greece | 9.5 |
| 43 | Canada | 8.3 |
| 44 | Cuba | 7.7 |
| 45 | Kuwait | 6.1 |
| 46 | USA | 5.7 |
| 47 | Sri Lanka | 3.7 |

Fig. 1

*Females,* 1981–1986

# AGE-STANDARDIZED DEATH RATES FOR STOMACH CANCER

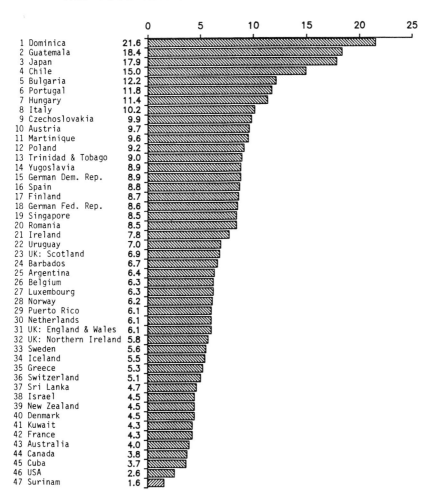

|    |                       |      |
|----|-----------------------|------|
| 1  | Dominica              | 21.6 |
| 2  | Guatemala             | 18.4 |
| 3  | Japan                 | 17.9 |
| 4  | Chile                 | 15.0 |
| 5  | Bulgaria              | 12.2 |
| 6  | Portugal              | 11.8 |
| 7  | Hungary               | 11.4 |
| 8  | Italy                 | 10.2 |
| 9  | Czechoslovakia        | 9.9  |
| 10 | Austria               | 9.7  |
| 11 | Martinique            | 9.6  |
| 12 | Poland                | 9.2  |
| 13 | Trinidad & Tobago     | 9.0  |
| 14 | Yugoslavia            | 8.9  |
| 15 | German Dem. Rep.      | 8.9  |
| 16 | Spain                 | 8.8  |
| 17 | Finland               | 8.7  |
| 18 | German Fed. Rep.      | 8.6  |
| 19 | Singapore             | 8.5  |
| 20 | Romania               | 8.5  |
| 21 | Ireland               | 7.8  |
| 22 | Uruguay               | 7.0  |
| 23 | UK: Scotland          | 6.9  |
| 24 | Barbados              | 6.7  |
| 25 | Argentina             | 6.4  |
| 26 | Belgium               | 6.3  |
| 27 | Luxembourg            | 6.3  |
| 28 | Norway                | 6.2  |
| 29 | Puerto Rico           | 6.1  |
| 30 | Netherlands           | 6.1  |
| 31 | UK: England & Wales   | 6.1  |
| 32 | UK: Northern Ireland  | 5.8  |
| 33 | Sweden                | 5.6  |
| 34 | Iceland               | 5.5  |
| 35 | Greece                | 5.3  |
| 36 | Switzerland           | 5.1  |
| 37 | Sri Lanka             | 4.7  |
| 38 | Israel                | 4.5  |
| 39 | New Zealand           | 4.5  |
| 40 | Denmark               | 4.5  |
| 41 | Kuwait                | 4.3  |
| 42 | France                | 4.3  |
| 43 | Australia             | 4.0  |
| 44 | Canada                | 3.8  |
| 45 | Cuba                  | 3.7  |
| 46 | USA                   | 2.6  |
| 47 | Surinam               | 1.6  |

number of populations should be regarded as minimum rates of incidence due to underascertainment of incident cancers and that a high gastric cancer ratio (ASCAR) may be due either to a high frequency of gastric cancer or to a low frequency of other types of cancer.

TABLE 1

AGE-STANDARDIZED INCIDENCE (ASIR) AND CUMULATIVE INCIDENCE RATES OF STOMACH CANCER

| Cancer Registry | Males | | Females | |
|---|---|---|---|---|
| | ASIR per 100,000 | Cumulative Rate (0-74 yrs) | ASIR per 100,000 | Cumulative Rate (0-74 yrs) |
| AMERICA | | | | |
| Costa Rica | 58.8 | 7.0 | 25.2 | 3.0 |
| Brazil - Sao Paulo | 53.6 | - | 25.1 | - |
| - Fortaleza | 44.6 | 5.5 | 16.7 | 2.1 |
| - Pto Alegre | 30.7 | - | 12.4 | - |
| - Recife | 29.9 | 3.7 | 8.6 | 1.0 |
| Colombia - Cali | 49.6 | 5.2 | 26.3 | 2.7 |
| Martinique | 25.3 | 2.9 | 10.9 | 1.4 |
| Netherlands Antilles | 19.1 | 2.3 | 7.1 | 0.8 |
| Puerto Rico | 17.6 | 2.0 | 8.6 | 1.0 |
| US Los Angeles: | | | | |
| - Korean | 44.8 | 7.8 | 18.6 | 2.2 |
| - Japanese | 25.5 | 2.7 | 11.4 | 1.1 |
| - Black | 15.6 | 1.8 | 6.4 | 0.8 |
| - Latino | 14.7 | 1.8 | 6.7 | 0.7 |
| - Chinese | 14.0 | 1.5 | 8.7 | 0.9 |
| - White | 8.6 | 1.0 | 4.0 | 0.4 |
| - Filipino | 4.7 | 0.6 | 2.6 | 0.4 |
| US Bay Area: | | | | |
| - Japanese | 24.3 | 2.7 | 10.8 | 1.0 |
| - Black | 19.1 | 2.2 | 6.0 | 0.6 |
| - White | 10.4 | 1.2 | 4.8 | 0.5 |
| - Chinese | 9.1 | 1.2 | 5.4 | 0.6 |
| - Filipino | 4.1 | 0.6 | 2.5 | 0.4 |

TABLE 1 continued

| Cancer Registry | Males ASIR per 100,000 | Cumulative Rate (0-74 yrs) | Females ASIR per 100,000 | Cumulative Rate (0-74 yrs) |
|---|---|---|---|---|
| US Hawaii: | | | | |
| - Hawaiian | 31.2 | 3.6 | 14.9 | 1.8 |
| - Japanese | 28.4 | 2.9 | 14.1 | 1.5 |
| - White | 11.8 | 1.3 | 6.0 | 0.6 |
| - Chinese | 11.2 | 1.2 | 6.7 | 0.6 |
| - Filipino | 6.8 | 0.6 | 4.6 | 0.4 |
| US Connecticut: | | | | |
| - Black | 19.4 | 2.2 | 9.1 | 1.1 |
| - White | 10.8 | 1.3 | 4.3 | 0.5 |
| US New Orleans: | | | | |
| - Black | 17.5 | 2.2 | 8.3 | 0.8 |
| - White | 7.3 | 0.8 | 3.2 | 0.4 |
| US Seattle | 8.0 | 0.9 | 3.3 | 0.4 |
| US Iowa | 6.8 | 0.8 | 3.0 | 0.3 |
| US Utah | 6.3 | 0.7 | 3.1 | 0.3 |
| Canada | 13.2 | 1.5 | 5.9 | 0.6 |
| - Newfoundland | 25.3 | 3.0 | 10.7 | 1.3 |
| - New Brunswick | 16.7 | 1.9 | 6.3 | 0.7 |
| - Quebec | 15.3 | 1.8 | 6.7 | 0.8 |
| - Alberta | 11.8 | 1.4 | 4.8 | 0.5 |
| - British Columbia | 11.9 | 1.4 | 5.0 | 0.5 |
| - NW Territories and Yukatan | 5.3 | 0.9 | 2.8 | 0.4 |
| ASIA | | | | |
| Japan - Nagasaki | 82.0 | 10.0 | 36 1 | 4.0 |
| - Hiroshima | 79.9 | 9.8 | 35.8 | 4.3 |
| - Miyagi | 79.6 | 9.7 | 36.0 | 4.2 |
| - Osaka | 76.9 | 9.1 | 35.9 | 4.0 |
| China - Shanghai | 58.3 | 7.4 | 24.6 | 3.0 |
| - Tianjin | 36.4 | 4.7 | 15.0 | 1.9 |
| Sigapore - Chinese | 37.3 | 4.6 | 15.4 | 1.8 |
| - Indian | 15.5 | 2.2 | 16.6 | 1.9 |
| - Malay | 9.4 | 1.3 | 6.8 | 0.8 |
| Hong Kong | 19.2 | 2.5 | 9.6 | 1.1 |

TABLE 1 continued

| Cancer Registry | Males | | Females | |
|---|---|---|---|---|
| | ASIR per 100,000 | Cumulative Rate (0-74 yrs) | ASIR per 100,000 | Cumulative Rate (0-74 yrs) |
| Israel: | | | | |
| - All Jews | 16.2 | 1.8 | 9.3 | 1.1 |
| - Born Europe/America | 18.3 | 2.0 | 10.3 | 1.1 |
| - Born Israel | 12.4 | 1.4 | 6.9 | 0.8 |
| - Born Africa/Asia | 12.3 | 1.5 | 7.2 | 0.9 |
| - Non Jews | 7.9 | 1.0 | 4.9 | 0.6 |
| India - Madras | 13.7 | 1.6 | 6.7 | 0.7 |
| - Bangalore | 12.6 | 1.5 | 7.1 | 0.7 |
| - Poona | 10.5 | 1.3 | 6.3 | 0.7 |
| - Bombay | 8.9 | 0.8 | 6.0 | 0.6 |
| - Nagpur | 7.8 | 0.9 | 6.7 | 0.8 |
| Philippines - Rizal | 9.4 | 1.1 | 6.7 | 0.7 |
| Kuwait - Non Kuwaitis | 8.7 | 1.0 | 3.9 | 0.5 |
| - Kuwaitis | 3.7 | 0.3 | 1.6 | 0.2 |
| OCEANIA | | | | |
| New Zealand | | | | |
| - Pac. Poly. Islands | 33.6 | 4.1 | 15.1 | 1.9 |
| - Maori | 29.8 | 4.2 | 19.7 | 2.4 |
| - Non Maori | 13.7 | 1.6 | 6.0 | 0.6 |
| Austalia - West | 15.1 | 1.7 | 5.0 | 0.6 |
| - Cap. Terr. | 15.0 | 1.7 | 6.4 | 0.6 |
| - South | 13.1 | 1.5 | 5.7 | 0.6 |
| - Tasmania | 12.6 | 1.6 | 4.8 | 0.5 |
| EUROPE | | | | |
| Italy - Parma | 44.0 | 4.5 | 19.9 | 2.1 |
| - Varese | 39.0 | 4.5 | 17.1 | 1.8 |
| - Ragusa | 19.8 | 2.3 | 8.4 | 0.7 |
| Poland - Nowy Sacz | 43.7 | 5.6 | 17.0 | 2.1 |
| - Cracow City | 32.9 | 4.0 | 13.4 | 1.6 |
| - Warsaw City | 23.2 | 2.8 | 8.9 | 1.0 |
| Yugoslavia - Slovenia | 34.9 | 4.4 | 15.1 | 1.7 |
| Romania - County Cluj | 34.2 | 4.2 | 13.6 | 1.7 |
| Hungary - Szabolcz | 32.4 | 4.1 | 12.8 | 1.5 |

TABLE 1 continued

| Cancer Registry | Males | | Females | |
|---|---|---|---|---|
| | ASIR per 100,000 | Cumulative Rate (0-74 yrs) | ASIR per 100,000 | Cumulative Rate (0-74 yrs) |
| Czechoslovakia - Slovakia | 31.7 | 3.9 | 14.5 | 1.7 |
| Spain - Navarra | 31.6 | 3.8 | 13.5 | 1.4 |
| - Zaragoza | 20.8 | 2.1 | 10.4 | 1.0 |
| - Tarragona | 16.9 | 1.9 | 7.8 | 0.8 |
| Iceland | 31.4 | 3.7 | 14.0 | 1.6 |
| German Democratic Republic | 25.2 | 3.1 | 12.3 | 1.4 |
| Finland | 24.6 | 2.8 | 12.9 | 1.4 |
| FR Germany - Hamburg | 23.7 | 2.6 | 11.7 | 1.3 |
| - Saarland | 23.6 | 2.7 | 12.1 | 1.2 |
| UK - England & Wales | 18.5 | 2.2 | 7.8 | 0.9 |
| - North Western | 22.0 | 2.7 | 9.8 | 1.1 |
| - East Scotland | 22.0 | 2.7 | 10.1 | 1.1 |
| - Oxford | 20.2 | 2.4 | 7.8 | 0.8 |
| - South Thames | 15.7 | 1.9 | 6.6 | 0.7 |
| - North Scotland | 14.7 | 1.9 | 6.2 | 0.8 |
| Netherlands - Eindhoven | 20.7 | 2.5 | 9.5 | 1.1 |
| Switzerland - Basel | 19.6 | 1.9 | 8.1 | 0.8 |
| - Neuchatel | 17.9 | 2.1 | 6.8 | 0.8 |
| - Vaud | 15.2 | 1.7 | 5.0 | 0.5 |
| - Geneva | 13.5 | 1.5 | 6.3 | 0.7 |
| Norway | 18.1 | 2.2 | 9.3 | 1.0 |
| France - Calvados | 15.8 | 2.0 | 8.1 | 0.9 |
| - Bas-Rhin | 15.5 | 1.9 | 7.4 | 0.9 |
| - Doubs | 15.2 | 1.8 | 6.7 | 0.8 |
| - Isere | 11.5 | 1.4 | 5.4 | 0.6 |
| Denmark | 14.3 | 1.6 | 6.7 | 0.7 |
| Ireland, Southern | 12.4 | 1.4 | 4.2 | 0.5 |

Rates adjusted to World Standard Population

From: Cancer Incidence in Five Continents, Vol. V (19)

TABLE 2

AGE-STANDARDIZED INCIDENCE RATES (ASIR) AND AGE-STANDARDIZED CANCER RATIOS (ASCAR) FOR STOMACH CANCER IN SELECTED POPULATIONS

| Cancer Registry | ASIR per 100,000 | |
|---|---|---|
| | Males | Females |
| **AFRICA** | | |
| Nigeria - Ibadan | 7.1 | 4.0 |
| Tanzania: | | |
| - Kilimanjaro | 5.6 | 4.6 |
| Senegal - Dakar* | 3.7 | 2.0 |
| Algeria - Algiers, | | |
| Oran & Constantine | 3.6 | 1.4 |
| Swaziland | 1.8 | 0.2 |
| **AMERICA** | | |
| Peru - Lima | 26.4 | 16.5 |
| Argentina - La Plata | 18.6 | 8.7 |
| Jamaica - Kingston* | 17.7 | 9.3 |
| Bolivia - La Paz | 13.9 | 10.3 |
| Cuba* | 12.4 | 6.6 |
| Paraguay | 12.1 | 5.7 |
| Panama | 9.9 | 6.2 |

| Cancer Registry | ASCAR (%) | |
|---|---|---|
| | Males | Females |
| **AFRICA** | | |
| Angola - Luanda | 15.0 | 7.2 |
| Rwanda - Nat. Reg. | 8.6 | 6.6 |
| Zambia - Lusaka | 6.3 | 4.7 |
| - Ndola | 0.5 | 2.8 |
| Kenya - Nat. Reg. | 6.0 | 3.9 |
| - Mombasa | 5.7 | 3.1 |
| Liberia | 4.2 | 1.7 |
| Uganda - Kampala | 2.9 | 2.1 |
| - West Nile | 1.0 | 0.0 |
| Malawi | 2.8 | 0.5 |
| Sudan | 2.6 | 2.7 |
| Tunisia | 2.6 | 1.9 |
| Madagascar | 1.9 | 0.6 |
| Gabon - Libreville | 0.8 | 1.8 |
| **ASIA** | | |
| Malaysia - Kuala Lumpur | 7.1 | 3.1 |
| Iraq - Baghdad | 5.3 | 4.4 |
| Bangladesh | 1.6 | 1.0 |
| Sri Lanka - Colombo | 1.2 | 0.5 |
| Vietnam: | | |
| - Ho Chi Minh City | 0.8 | 0.2 |

From: "Cancer Occurrence in Developing Countries" (25) except for registries marked with an asterisk, for which the data comes from "Cancer Incidence in Five Continents, Vol. IV" (32).

The high rates in Japan, China, Costa Rica, Brazil, Colombia, Koreans in Los Angeles, North Italy, Poland, Yugoslavia, Romania, Hungary, Czechoslovakia, North Spain, Iceland, Polynesians and Maoris in New Zealand, and the relatively low rates and ratios for most African populations are the most noteworthy features of Table 1 and 2. In Japan, the cumulative rate for the age group 0-74 years is about 10% in males, indicating that 10% of Japanese males who do not die from other causes and reach the age of 74 will develop stomach cancer. The equivalent rate is shown as less than 1% for African populations in Vols III and IV of "Cancer Incidence in Five Continents" (31,32), about 1% in India, the Philippines and Caucasian populations in North American and Oceania, and it ranges from 2-5% in Europe and between 5-8% in some Latin American countries, China and Koreans in the USA.

## Distribution by Sex and Age

In most populations shown in Tables 1 and 2 and Figures 1 and 2, there is a two- to three-fold excess of stomach cancer in males, except in Guatemala, Sri Lanka, Bolivia and Tanzania, where the sex ratio is less than or close to one. In the USA, migrants from high-risk countries display higher rates than the native population, and blacks have a two-fold increase over whites. In all populations, gastric cancer is extremely rare below the age of 30; thereafter, it increases rapidly and steadily to reach the highest rates in the oldest age groups, both in males and females. The increase with age is less steep, however, when age-specific rates are plotted for successive birth cohorts both in populations at both high and low risk for gastric cancer (12).

As mentioned above, in most populations the sex ratio of the age-adjusted rates is about 2-3 but, when the age-specific rates are considered, a variation of this ratio with age emerged, as originally described by Griffiths (7). Below the age of 30, the sex ratio is close to one, it then increases to reach a maximum in the age group 55-59, and thereafter declines progressively (7).

## Intra-country Variation

Tables 1 and 2 and Figures 1 and 2 give an up-to-date general view of the frequency of stomach cancer around the world, but they contain limited information on the remarkable variation in frequency within relatively small areas. National data on intra-country differences hae recently been reviewed (12). A north-south gradient in gastric cancer rates has been observed in several countries such as the USA, Japan, China, England and Wales, Yugoslavia, Italy, Spain and Ireland (12). In Latin American countries, however, the gradient is the reverse or does not exist. In Colombia, a higher risk of gastric cancer has been described in the south in the Andean department of Narino than in the central valleys and Atlantic coast (4). In Brazil, no clear gradient is apparent: higher rates are reported from the cancer registries of Sao Paulo in the south and Fortalesa in the north-east, than from Porto

Alegre in the south and Recife in the north-east (see Table 1). In Costa Rica, the highest rates are observed in the highland area in the centre of the country and the lowest rates in the peripheral coastal areas (18,29).

It is interesting to note that in Colombia and Costa Rica, it has been shown that the prevalence of precancerous lesions of the stomach, ie chronic atrophic gastritis and intestinal metaplasia is also higher in the high-risk areas than in the low-risk areas for gastric cancer (4,10,28,29).

Urban-rural distribution

Table 3 give the age adjusted incidence rates in urban and rural populations for those cancer registries which provided these data to Vo. V of "Cancer Incidence in Five Continents" (19). It does not show important or consistent gradients in risk between urban and rural populations. However, in countries such as Colombia and Costa Rica, which show large differences in risk within relatively small areas, most of the high-risk populations are from rural areas. The rates for cities, which have a heavy influx of migrants, should be considered as a weighted average of the rates of the native and migrant populations, as suggested by Correa et al (4).

TABLE 3

AGE-STANDARDIZED INCIDENCE RATES (ASIR) OF STOMACH CANCER: URBAN-RURAL DISTRIBUTION

| Cancer Registry | ASIR per 100,000 | |
| --- | --- | --- |
| | Urban | Rural |
| Japan - Mayagi | 79.2 | 80.1 |
| Romania - Country Cluj | 32.6 | 35.7 |
| Hungary - Szabolcz | 32.6 | 32.5 |
| Czechoslovakia - Slovakia | 29.9 | 32.0 |
| FR Germany - Saarland | 24.5 | 21.4 |
| UK - England and Wales | 18.9 | 15.0 |
| France - Doubs | 16.4 | 13.1 |
| - Calvados | 15.2 | 16.9 |
| Norway | 18.5 | 17.8 |
| Switzerland - Vaud | 14.3 | 15.8 |

From: Cancer Incidence in Five Continents, Vol V (19)

Time Trends

A steady decrease in stomach cancer rates has been apparent in most populations since the early decades of this century. Figure 3 taken from a recent publication (15) shows the time trends for 24 countries for the period 1950-51 to 1978-79. The steady decline is apparent for all countries in both sexes. In high-risk countries such as Japan, Chile and Portugal the decline has occurred later than in low-risk countries such as the USA. A closer look of the time trends in Norway shows that mortality rates started to decline in 1930, levelled off during the 1940-45 war and reassumed its decline in 1951 (Figure 4). Dietary changes occurring during the war, involving mainly a decrease in fat intake, specially milk fat, and an increase in cereal intake, correlated well with the gastric cancer trend (20). Although a large number of hypotheses have been proposed to explain the decline in stomach cancer in most populations, the actual factors responsible for it remain unrevealed.

Social Class and Occupation

An inverse socio-economic gradient has been observed in most populations, the rate in lower socio-economic groups being two to three times higher than in more affluent classes (8,30). An excess risk has been linked to certain occupations such as coal mining, fishing and agriculture (9). Since occupations are clearly related to socio-economic backgorund, some of the excess risk observed might be attributable to patterns of lifestyle such as dietary habits.

Risk in Migrant Populations

Several epidemiological studies of migrants to the USA, have shown that migrant born in high-risk countries retain their high risk when they move to the low-risk environment of the USA (8,10). However, their US-born offspring show rates closer to those of the adopted country. Table 4 gives the age-adjusted rates for Chinese and Japanese populations in their native countries and the adopted countries as shown in Vol. V of "Cancer Incidence in Five Continents" (19). The exact interpretation of these rates is difficult if we consider that in both China and Japan there are marked intra-country variations in the rates for Japanese and Chinese migrants to the USA represent the rates for both the first and second generations of migrants. Despite these difficulties, a general, pattern is apparent: The stomach cancer rates for Japanese and Chinese living int he USA are intermediate between those of their host countries and those of the adopted country.

Studies in migrants have helped enormously in understanding the dynamics of stomach cancer and its precursor lesions. They provide clear evidence of the critical importance of exposures in early life in determining the risk of developing, as a first stage, the precancerous lesions and, subsequently, stomach cancer.

Epidemiology of the Two Main Histological Types of Gastric Cancer

Two main histological types of gastric cancer, which differ not only in morphology but also in their epdiemiological characteristics, have been described.

62

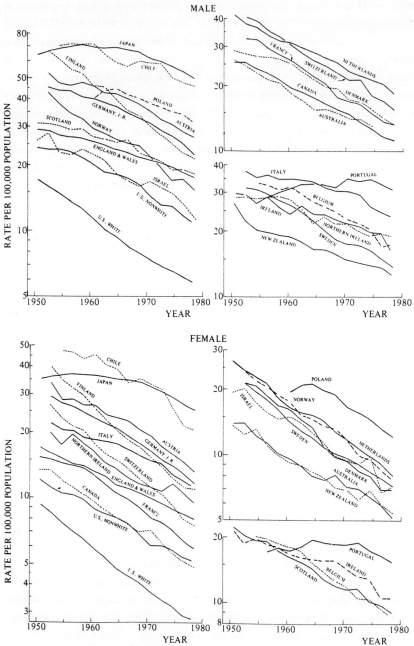

Fig. 3    Trends in age-adjusted death rates for malignant neoplasm of stomach from 1950-51 to 1978-79 in 24 countries

TABLE 4

AGE-STANDARDIZED INCIDENCE RATES (ASIR) OF STOMACH CANCER IN NATIVE AND MIGRANT
POPULATIONS

| | ASIR per 100,000 | | | ASCAR (%) | |
| | Males | Females | | Males | Females |
|---|---|---|---|---|---|
| Japanese | | | Chinese | | |
| Living in: | | | Living in: | | |
| Japan (Nagasaki) | 82.0 | 36.1 | China (Shanghai) | 58.3 | 24.6 |
| Japan (Osaka) | 76.9 | 35.9 | China (Tianjin) | 36.4 | 15.0 |
| US Bay Area | 24.3 | 10.8 | Hong Kong | 19.2 | 9.6 |
| US Los Angeles | 25.5 | 11.4 | Singapore | 37.3 | 15.4 |
| US Hawaii | 28.4 | 14.1 | US Los Angeles | 14.0 | 8.7 |
| US Whites | | | US Bay Area | 9.1 | 5.4 |
| Living in: | | | US Hawaii | 11.2 | 6.7 |
| Bay Area | 10.4 | 4.8 | Other Ethnic Groups | | |
| Los Angeles | 8.6 | 4.0 | Living in Singapore: | | |
| Hawaii | 11.8 | 6.0 | Indian | 15.5 | 16.6 |
| | | | Malay | 9.4 | 6.8 |

From: "Cancer Incidence in Five Continents, Vol. V" (19)

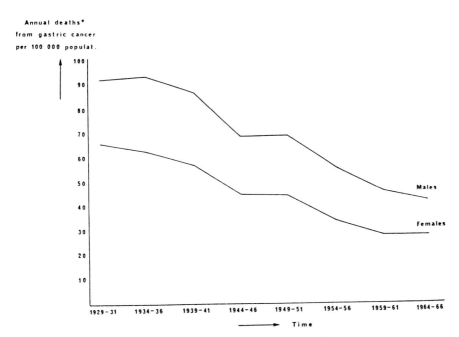

Lauren proposed the original classifciation into "intestinal" for those tumours which morphologically resemble the colonic mucosa, and "diffuse" for those carcinomas which diffusely infiltrate the gastric wall (16). Later on, Ming proposed the terms of "expanding" for the former and "infiltrative" for the latter (17). About 10-20% of tumours cannot be assigned to either group and these were called "others". The intestinal or expanding type is characterized by the tendency to form glandular structures with an intestinal appearance and has often, grossly, a polypoid appearance. It is more prevalent in males and older age groups. The diffuse or infiltrative type is characterized by lack of cellular cohesiveness and diffuse infiltration of the gastric wall, its sex ratio is closer to one, it is relatively more frequent in younger age groups, and it has a worse prognosis than the intestinal type.

Below, I will describe the prinicpal epidemiological characteristics of these two types of stomach cancer:

Geographical distribution. Table 5 summarizes some studies giving the distribution of the two main types of stomach cancer in high-, intermediate- and low-risk popultions in Colombia, Yugoslavia, Poland, Mexico and the UK. The age-standarized incidence rates are given for time periods as close as possible to those for which the histological material was reviewed. For Cali (Colombia) and Yugoslavia (Slovenia) from "Cancer Incidence in Five Continents, Vol. II" (6) for Poland (Katowice) from "Cancer Incidence in Five Continents, Vol. III" (31); for the UK, the rates were obtained form reports of the cancer registries of North Wales (27) and East Anglia (1), respectively, for Cartagena from a previous publication (22) and for Barranquilla and Mexico the incidence rates were estimated from mortality rates.

All histological slides from the various countries, except those of England, were reviewed by the author of this paper using Lauren's classification. Detailed results have been published elsewhere (2,3,22,23). In one of the original reports, age-adjusted incidence rates were estimated for the two types of Cali and Cartagena in Colombia and in Finland, and it was concluded that most of the excess gastric cancer risk in Cali and Finland could be accounted for by an excess in the intestinal type (22). In both North Wales and Norfolk, there were pockets with a high intestinal/diffuse ratio (2,3).

Although these findings do not agree with those reported by Kubo (13,14), his use of different classification criteria may explain some of the differences.

Age Distribution and Sex Ratio. Differences have been described in the age distribution curves of the two types of gastric cancer and between those of males and females: the risk for the intestinal type rises faster with age than the risk for the diffuse type, both in high- and low-risk populations, and for females the rise for intestinal type occurs at older ages than for males (5). This male/female difference

TABLE 5

HISTOLOGICAL TYPES OF GASTRIC CANCER IN HIGH- AND LOW-RISK POPULATIONS

| | ASIR* per 100,000 | Total Cases | Histological Types (%) | | | Ratio Intestinal/ Diffuse |
|---|---|---|---|---|---|---|
| | | | Intestinal | diffuse | Others | |
| **High-risk areas** | | | | | | |
| Colombia - Cali (22) | 57.5 | 191 | 51.8 | 34.0 | 14.1 | 1.5 |
| Yugoslavia - Maribor (23) | 46.1 | 149 | 51.7 | 34.8 | 13.4 | 1.5 |
| Poland - Gliwice (23) | 36.0 | 94 | 45.7 | 36.2 | 18.1 | 1.3 |
| UK - North Wales (2) | 43.0 | 490 | 54.1 | 23.5 | 22.4 | 2.3 |
| TOTAL | | 924 | 52.5 | 28.8 | 18.7 | 1.8 |
| **Intermediat-risk areas** | | | | | | |
| UK - Norfolk and Norwich (3) | 27.4 | 252 | 61.1 | 25.0 | 13.9 | 2.4 |
| - Gorleston (3) | | 120 | 77.5 | 10.0 | 12.5 | 7.8 |
| TOTAL | | 372 | 66.4 | 20.2 | 13.4 | 3.3 |
| **Low-risk areas** | | | | | | |
| Colombia - Cartagena (22) | 12.2 | 38 | 28.9 | 53.3 | 15.8 | 0.5 |
| - Barranquilla (22) | 10.0 | 13 | 38.5 | 46.1 | 15.4 | 0.8 |
| Mexico - Mexico City (22) | 7.0 | 80 | 38.7 | 46.3 | 15.0 | 0.8 |
| Yugoslavia - Koper (23) | | 53 | 39.6 | 50.9 | 9.5 | 0.8 |
| TOTAL | | 184 | 37.0 | 49.4 | 13.6 | 0.7 |

*Rates adjusted to the World Standard Population

From:  Munoz et al (22)
Munoz and Matko (23)
Caygill et al (2)
Caygill et al (3)

ESTIMATED AGE AND SEX SPECIFIC DEATH RATES
PER 100,000 OF INTESTINAL TYPE OF GASTRIC CANCER

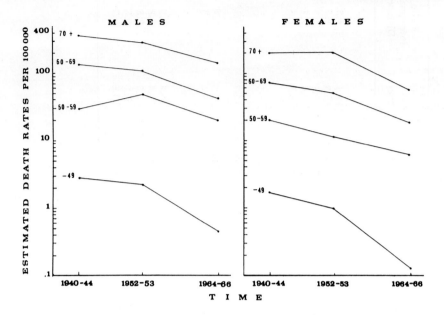

ESTIMATED AGE AND SEX DEATH RATES PER
1000,000 OF DIFFUSE TYPE OF GASTRIC
CANCER

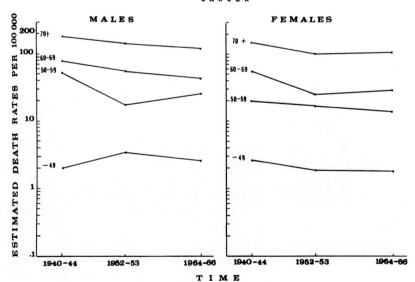

would explain the peak of the sex ratio in the age group 55-59, as originally described by Griffith (7).

Urban-rural Distribution. A predominance of the intestinal type has been described in rural areas of England. Caygill et al (2,3) reported in intestinal/diffuse ratio of 2.4 in coastal and urban areas and of 4.8 in inland and rural areas of North Wales. similar observations were made earlier in Colombia (4).

Time Trends. In Norway the time trends for the two main types of gastric cancer were studied using random samples of most of the gastric cancers diagnosed in the whole country for three time periods: 1940-44, 1952-53 and 1964-66. Figures 5 and 6 show that most of the decline in gastric cancer occurring from the second to the third period could be explained by a decline in the intestinal type, especially in the age groups under 50 (20). Similar tendencies have been reported in the USA (21) and in a population-based study in Osaka, Japan (11). In the UK, although no significant difference in the distribution of the two types was observed between 1940-46 and 1971-73, the intestinal/diffuse ratio decreased from 3.2 in the first period to 1.6 in the second (33). However, the number of cases included in this study, specially in the second time period (22 cases), is too small to draw meaningful conclusions.

Migrant Studies. In Israel, a predominance of intestinal type was observed in migrants from high-risk countries (mainly Eastern-Europe) but not in those from low-risk countries. The intestinal/diffuse ratio in migrants from high-risk countries was 2.0, and it was 0.9 in migrants from low-risk countries (24). Correa et al (4) studied the prevalence of the two types of gastric cancer and its precursor lesions among internal migrants in Colombia. The risks for gastric cancer in each migrant group to the city of Cali reflected well the levels found in their native home. Correa et al (5) also compared age-specific and type-specific incidence rates of gastric cancer among Japanese living in Miyagi, Japan (high-risk area) and Japanese who had migrated to the low-risk area of Hawaii. They concluded that most of the decline in gastric cancer rates of the Japanese migrants to Hawaii could be explained by a decline in the intestinal type, since the incidence of the diffuse type remained unchanged.

CONCLUSION

The descriptive epdiemiology of stomach cancer is characterized by: the existence of large regional differences within relatively small geographic confines, even in small countries with relatively homogeneous populations such as Costa Rica, a marked and steady decline in all populations, the cirtical role of exposures in early life in determining the risk, as suggsted by migrant studies. All these observations strongly suggest that the major determinants of gastric cancer, and specifically the

68

intestinal type, are environmental rather than genetic. Although the major causes of stomach cancer remain unknown, a large number of aetiological hypotheses incriminating several environmental and lifestyle variable have been proposed, and most of these will be reviewed at this symposium, together with the influence of genetic factors.

REFERENCES

1.   Annual Report of the Cancer Registration Bureau of the East Anglia Region, year 1982-83, pp 29

2.   Caygill C, Day DW, Hill MJ (1983) Br J Cancer 48:603-605

3.   Caygill C, Day DW, Hill MJ (1986) Br J Cancer 53:145-147

4.   Correa P, Cuello C, Duque E et al (1970) J Natl Cancer Inst 44:297-306

5.   Correa P, Sasano N, Stemmermann N et al (1973) J Natl Cancer Inst 51:1449-1459

6.   Doll R, Muir C, Waterhouse J (eds) (1970) Cancer Incidence in Five Continents, Vol. II. International Union Against Cancer, Geneva

7.   Griffith GW (1968) Br J Cancer 22:163-172

8.   Haenszel W (1958) J Natl Cancer Inst 21:213-262

9.   Haenszel W. Correa P (1975) Cancer Res 35:3452-3459

10.  Haenszel W, Kurihara M (1968) J Natl Cancer Inst 40:43-68

11.  Hanai A, Fujimoto I, Taniguchi H (1982) In: Magnus K (ed) Trends in Cancer Incidence: Causes and Practical Implicatons. Hemisphere Publ corp, New York, pp143-154

12.  Howson CP, Hiyama T, Wynder EL (1986) Epidemiol Rev 8:1-27

13.  Kubo T (1971) Cancer 28:726-734

14.  Kubo T (1973) Cancer 31:1498-1507

15.  Kurihara M, Aoki K, tominaga S (eds) (1984) Cancer Mortality Statistics in the World. University of Nagoya Press, Nagoya

16.  Lauren P (1965) Acta Pathol Microbiol Scand 64:31-49

17.  Ming SC (1977) Cancer 39:2475-2485

18.  Miranda M, Macay I, Moya L (1977) Acta Medica Costaricense 20:207-214

19.  Muir C, Waterhouse J, Mack T, Powell J, Whelan S (eds) (1987) Cancer Incidence in five Continents, Vol. V, IARC Sci Publ No 88. International Agency for Research on Cancer, Lyon.

20.  Munoz N, Asvall J (1971) Int J Cancer 8:144-157

21.  Munoz N, Connely R (1971) Int J Cancer 8:158-164

22.  Munoz N, Correa P, Cuello C, Duque E (1968) Int J Cancer 3:809-818

23.  Munoz N, Matko I (1972) Recent Results in Cancer Research 48:603-605

24.  Munoz N, Steinitz R (1971) Israel J Med Sci 7:1479-1487

25.  Parkin DM (ed) (1986) Cancer Occurrence in Developing Countries, IARC Sci Publ No 75. International Agency for Research on Cancer, Lyon

26.  Parkin DM, Laara E, Muir CS (1988) Int J Cancer 41:184-197

27.    Report of the Mersey Regional Cancer Registry, 1974-77.

28.    Salas I (1977) Patologia 15:63-79

29.    Sierra R, Parkin DM, Barrantes R, Bieber A, Munoz G, Munoz N (1988) Cancer in Costa Rica. IARC Technical Report No 1.    International Agency for Research on Cancer, Lyon, pp13-16

30.    Teppo L, Pukkala E, Hakama M et al (1980) Scand J Soc Med (Suppl) 19:1-84

31.    Waterhouse J, Muir C, Correa P, Powell J (eds) (1976) Cancer Incidence in Five Continents, Vol. III, IARC Sci Publ No 15. International Agency for Research on Cancer, Lyon

32.    Waterhouse J, Muir C, Shanmugaratnam K, Powell J (eds) (1982) Cancer Incidence in Five Continents, Vol. IV, IARC Sci Publ No 42. International Agency for Research on Cancer, Lyon

33.    Whitehead R, Skinner JM, Heenan PJ (1974) Br J Cancer 30:270-372

34.    World Health Organization (1987) World Health Statistics Annual. WHO, Geneva

© *Elsevier Science Publishers B.V. (Biomedical Division)*
*Gastric carcinogenesis. P.I. Reed, M.J. Hill, editors.*

## ACHLORHYDRIA AND CARCINOID TUMOURS

K G WORMSLEY
Ninewells Hospital, Dundee DD1 9SY, UK

The recent development of powerful gastric secretory inhibitors has focussed attention on a previously unemphasised association between gastric secretory failure and proliferative abnormalities of the gastric mucosa. More than 10 powerful gastric secretory inhibitors have produced achlorhydria in animals and man and have also produced proliferation of the gastric mucosa (of animals), resulting ultimately in frank neoplastic transformation (58).

These observations have raised an interesting set of problems: Are the proliferative abnormalities primary and the cause of the achlorhydria? Or does the achlorhydria somehow 'cause' the proliferative abnormalities of the gastric mucosa? Or are both achlohydria and mucosal proliferation caused by some common underlying mechanisms?

## ARE THE PROLIFERATIVE ABNORMALITIES OF THE GASTRIC MUCOSA THE CAUSE OF THE ACHLORHYDRIA?

It has long been recognised that conditions which are assumed to be primarily proliferative disorders of the gastric mucosa (such as chronic atrophic gastritis, or pernicious anaemia) result in achlorhydria. It has further been assumed that the gastric secretory failure is the direct consequence of the disturbance of proliferation and differentiation of the precursor cells of the gastric mucosa, which have resulted in the production of mucus-producing cells and intestinal-type mucosa instead of acid-secreting parietal cells and pepsin-producing chief cells. The increased likelihood of developing adenocarcinomatous change in these proliferatively abnormal mucosae has been convincingly documented (13,36,54). It has also been noted that, rarely, the neoplastic end-point of the mucosal proliferation manifests morphologically as 'endocrine cell tumours' (carcinoids) (8,43,48).

Surprisingly, no enquiries appear to have been made regarding the nature and cause of the mucosal proliferative abnormalities, perhaps in part because 'gastritis' is still considered to be an 'inflammation' rather than a proliferative disorder. However, assuming that the gastric mucosa in chronic atrophic gastritis and in pernicious anaemia represents primarily a disturbance of proliferation of the precursor cells of the gastric mucosa, it is a necessary consequence that failure to produce specialised parietal cells results in achlorhydria. That the proliferative abnormalities also culminate in frank malignancy is both coincidental and also connected with the achlorhydria. Thus, the gastric carcinogenesis in patients with gastric mucosal disease is assumed to reflect an interaction between the abnormal proliferation of the gastric mucosal cells and the effects of intraluminally produced genotoxic carcinogens (13,14,27).

It has been proposed that, as in other cases of 'multistage' carcinogenesis, the abnormally proliferating cells 'fix', and permit the preferential expression of mutations produced by genotoxic carcinogens. The gastric mucosal cells in chronic atrophic gastritis and in pernicious anaemia already show evidence of altered expression of the DNA of the precursor cells (in the form of abnormal proliferation and abnormal development into phenotypical mucous and intestinal cells). It is therefore assumed that, like other transformed cells (5,16,37,44), these phenotypically abnormal cells are more likely to mutate further in the progression to malignancy. The nongenotoxic aspect of carcinogenesis in diseases such as pernicious anaemia is therefore independent of the coincident achlorhydria although, interestingly, many of the same pathophysiological conditions which are considered to be causally important in drug-induced gastric carcinogenesis are also present in pernicious anaemia, but are not considered relevant in the carcinogenesis associated with the latter disease.

On the other hand, the genotoxic carcinogens involved in the development of gastric cancer in chronic atrophic gastritis and pernicious anaemia are mainly considered to arise as a direct consequence of the achlorhydria. It has often been proposed that achlorhydria results in bacterial overgrowth in the gastric contents. The bacteria include nitrate-reducing genera, which reduce dietary and salivary nitrate to nitrite. The resulting nitrite is then converted to oxides of nitrogen which are assumed to react with intraluminally available amine groups to form carcinogenic N-nitroso compounds (13,39). A number of these assumptions and steps of 'logic' are, as yet, unfounded. For example, it is not possible for nitrosation to occur as described above because the physico-chemical conditions in the absence of free hydrogen ions do not permit the formation of nitrous acid and nitrogen oxides (22,23). While it is possible that nitrosation may occur as a result of the direct effect of nitrate reducing bacteria (11,32), no such production of N-nitroso compounds has been demonstrated in patients in vivo. It is true that the concentration of N-nitroso compounds (and of other food borne gastric carcinogens) is increased in the gastric contents of patients with chronic atrophic gastritis and with pernicious anaemia (40,45), at least in part because no diluting gastric juice is secreted. It is also likely that an increased concentration of N-nitroso compounds (and other carcinogens) in the environment of the gastric mucosal cells is more likely to be damaging than a 'normal' concentration, although no information is available about the tissue toxicity of the gastric intraluminal carcinogens found in these patients (28,46).

In view of the interest and importance attached to the apparent 'endocrine cell' hyperplasia and neoplasia associated with drug-induced achlorhydria, it is extraordinary that so little attention has been paid to the phenotypic manifestation of the malignant tumours found in patients with chronic atrophic gastritis and pernicious anaemia. No estimate has been provided of the relative proportion of adenocarcinomas to other neoplasms, such as carcinoids and lymphomas, probably because adenocarcinomas and derivatives are so much more common than other morphological variants. In this connection, it is necessary to emphasise that the phenotypic (morphological) manifestation of any malignant tumour depends on the activated normal and abnormal genes which are expressed in the affected malignant tissue (37). The human gastric mucosa is exposed to a large variety of potential genotoxic carcinogens and it is therefore not surprising that the cancers which ultimately develop are malignant, rather than benign (having been subjected to more "multi-hits" (44) than, for example, the gastric mucosa of experimental animals provided with regulated diets and living under sterilised laboratory conditions). Even so, the human gastric cancers are often morphologically 'mixed', showing glandular and endocrine cells (1,7,10,49) and sometimes even cells with both exocrine and endocrine features (12,25).

Summarising. In gastric mucosal disease, the achlorhydria is assumed to be secondary to the mucosal disease but the achlorhydria participates indirectly in the development of the gastric cancers which characterise chronic atrophic gastritis and pernicious anaemia.

## DOES THE ACHLORHYDRIA CAUSE THE PROLIFERATIVE ABNORMALITIES?

While it seems unlikely that achlorhydria is primary and 'causes' the mucosal changes associated with pernicious anaemia, no information is actually available about the nature of the changes which precede the development of pernicious anaemia, so that at present no definitive conclusions are possible about the chronological sequence of the association between achlorhydria and pernicious anaemia. Conversely, it has been shown that there are conditions, such as the WDHA syndrome (17) and patients with the Zollinger-Ellison syndrome in whom treatment has been discontinued (50), in which achlorhydria is associated with apparently normal gastric mucosal morphology, including normal (or increased) numbers of parietal cells.

Currently, the topic which is causing maximal controversy concerns the relationship between drug-induced achlorhydria and the development of gastric carcinoids. The hypothesis which enjoys current popularity proposes that the gastric inhibitory drugs produce achlorhydria which, in turn, elicits hypergastrinaemia, the latter stimulating hyperplasia and neoplastic change in the gastric fundic endocrine cells (21,30). I have previously discussed this hypothesis in detail and found each of the assumptions flawed (59).

Chronologically the achlorhydria precedes the proliferative abnormalities, even though mitotic activity of the fundic ECL cells is observed as early as 48 hours after administration of the gastric secretory inhibitor omeprazole (56). Treatment with omeprazole also increases secretion of gastrin within 2 hours and increases the production of gastrin mRNA within 24 hours (9).

What might be the link between achlorhydria and mucosal cellular proliferation? It has been proposed that achlorhydria-induced hypergastrinaemia is the operational link between drugs and gastric mucosal proliferation. I have previously discussed the lack of evidence for the assumption that achlorhydria stimulates release of gastrin (59). Worse, the effect of hypergastrinaemia on gastric cellular proliferation has not been tested directly because the effects of giving abnormally large amounts of gastrin for prolonged periods of time have not been studied. Administration of pentagastrin in rats has been reported to increase the proportion of endocrine cells in the gastric glands (6) but unfortunately the mitogenic effects of pentagastrin differ from those of gastrin. Many studies have shown that conditions which give rise to hypergastrinaemia also result in gastric mucosal (and especially endocrine cell) hyperplasia (18,20). While the latter association may indeed indicate that hypergastinaemia provides the mitogenic stimulus for the gastric mucosal proliferation, it is also possible that the hypergastrinaemia illustrates the finding that many different types of endocrine cell proliferate in response to treatment with gastric secretory inhibitors.

Indeed, it is not only the gastric fundic ECL cells which proliferate after administration of gastric secretory inhibitors. Within a few hours of the administration of omeprazole, the number of G cells in the antral mucosa has increased significantly (2,31). Since the duration between the exposure to gastric secretory inhibitors and the increase in the number of G cells was too short to be explained by replication of the G cells, it was proposed that G cells, previously invisible (using current techniques for identification) or unrecognisable as G cells, had transformed into the morphological G cells (31). The latter hypothesis raises all sorts of interesting problems, but it is acknowledged that peptide-exporting cells can change their product with what may be dramatic functional results in, for example, paracrine function. Moreover, while morphological changes reflect functional changes in peptide secreting cells, the altered cells may no longer be subject to the same functional controls as 'normal' cells. It seems possible, therefore, that the increased secretion of gastrin reflects abnormal 'autonomous' function of these newly apparent G cells. In this connection, it has also been reported that gastric carcinoids may produce gastrin (42).

The matter may be even more complex. As suggested previously (59), if the proliferating endocrine cells of the gastric fundic mucosa secrete a trophic peptide such as bombesin or GRP, as do the proliferating endocrine cells of the bronchial mucosa (33,35), the latter peptide may be responsible not only for the hypergastrinaemia, but also for the G cell hyperplasia. Even more interestingly, in addition to producing inappropriate peptides, abnormally proliferating endocrine cells may be susceptible to the mitogenic effects of the secreted peptide, resulting perhaps in an 'autocrine' stimulus to growth (as is seen in the small cell carcinomas of the bronchial mucosa, which secrete and are stimulated to proliferate by GRP (15,57)).

There are further, indirect means by which achlorhydria could stimulate gastric mucosal proliferation. It has been shown that genotoxic nitrosamines, applied to the bronchial mucosa, can produce endocrine cell hyperplasia and carcinoids (41). It is necessary to exclude the possibility, therefore, that either the secretory inhibitors are directly acting as mitogens or that the achlorhydria has resulted in intragastric or intraalimentary conditions which permit the production of gastrotoxic N-nitroso compounds. In man, treatment with omeprazole for 4 weeks was accompanied by increased concentrations of N-nitroso compounds in only a proportion of treated individuals (47).

ARE BOTH ACHLORHYDRIA AND GASTRIC MUCOSAL PROLIFERATION PRODUCED BY SOME COMMON, UNDERLYING MECHANISM?

It has recently been shown that omeprazole and some $H_2$ receptor antagonists stimulate hypergastrinaemia directly, while other $H_2$ receptor antagonists do not (38). It is not known whether the latter property of the gastric secretory inhibitors is related to the mitogenic effects of gastric secretory inhibition. However, two small pointers exist which suggest that omeprazole may exert direct effects on the proliferation of gastric endocrine cells. Thus, it was shown some years ago that omeprazole increases the number of ECL cells in the gastric mucosa of antrectomised rats (53) despite the development of atrophic gastritis after antrectomy (19,34). Moreover, it has been stated that there is no significant hypergastrinaemia at the time (48 hours after administration) that ECL cells start proliferating (56). Similarly, it has been reported that a new $H_2$ receptor antagonist produces ECL cell hyperplasia in doses which do not give rise to hypergastrinaemia (26). While these findings imply the possibility of a direct mitogenic effect of the drug, it has been argued that in the latter two studies, diurnal variations in the levels of circulating gastrin were not studied and that hypergastrinaemia, occurring during part of the day could have escaped detection and yet have exerted mitogenic effects.

Other $H_2$ receptor antagonists have exerted what seem to be direct genotoxic effects on the gastric mucosa. For example, tiotidine has produced antral carcinomas similar to those produced by MNNG (51,52), while an even more interesting reaction has been produced by the $H_2$ receptor antagonist SK and F 93479. The latter drug not only produced squamous cell carcinomas of the forestomach of rats, but also produced endocrine cell hyperplasia and carcinoids of the fundic mucosa (3,4,24). As with MNNG-induced experimental cancer of the stomach (29,55), it seems that the morphological expression of the resulting cancer is independent of the cells of origin of the cancer, since both epithelial and neuro-endocrine components of the neoplasms can be derived from common precursor cells.

## SUMMARY

The attention which has been paid to the association between achlorhydria and carcinoids is too recent to permit more than speculation about the nature of the association. In man, it is not known to what extent achlorhydria is associated with the development of carcinoid tumours, even in patients (like those with pernicious anaemia) who suffer from gastric mucosal disease. Moreover, carcinoid tumours do occur in the stomach of patients without gastric mucosal disease (24) and who are, therefore, presumably not achlorhydric. Until the many different facets of achlorhydira, gastric inhibitory drugs and gastric mucosal disease have been better defined, a plea is made that facile oversimplifications of the nature of the association between these factors be avoided.

## REFERENCES

1. Ambe K, Mori M, Enjoji M (1987) Am J Surg Pathol 11: 310-315

2. Arnold R, Koop H, Schwarting H, Tuch K, Willemer B (1986) Scand J Gastroenterol 21: Suppl 125, 14-19

3. Betton GR, Harleman JH, Salmon GK (1987) Toxicology 6: 4

4. Betton GR, Salmon GK (1984) Scand J Gastroenterol 19: Suppl 101, 103-108

5. Bishop JM (1987) Science 235: 305-311

6. Blom H (1986) Digestion 35: Suppl 1, 98-105

7. Bonar SF, Sweeney EC (1986) Histopathology 10: 53-63

8. Borch K, Renvall H, Liedberg G (1986) Digestion 35: suppl 1, 106-115

9. Brand SJ, Stone D (1987) Gastroenterology 92: 1326

10. Burtin P, Cerez H, Simeliere T, Ben Bouali A, d'Aubigny N, Person B, Boyer J (1987) Ann Gastroenterol Hepatol 23: 251-256

11. Camels S, Ohshima H, Rosenkranz H, McCoy E, Bartsch H (1987) Carcinogenesis 8: 1085-1088

12. Chejfec G, Capella C, Solcia E, Jao W, Gould VE (1985) Cancer 56: 2683-2690

13. Correa P (1983) Cancer Surv 2: 437-450

14. Correa P (1985) In: Joosens JV, Hill MJ, Geboers J (eds) Diet and human carcinogenesis. Excerpta Medica, Amsterdam, pp109-115

15. Cuttitta F, Carney DN, Mulshine J, Moody TW, Fedorko J, Fischler A, Minna JD (1985) Nature 316: 823-826

16. Farber E (1984) Cancer Res 44: 5463-5474

17. Gjone E, Fretheim B, Nordoy A, Jacobsen CD, Elgjo K (1970) Scand J Gastroenterol 5: 401-408

18. Hakanson R, Blom H, Carlsson E, Larsson H, Ryberg B, Sundler F (1986) Regulatory Peptides 13: 225-233

19. Hakanson R, Larsson LI, Liedberg G, Oscarson J, Sundler F, Vang J (1976) J Physiol 259: 785-800

20. Hakanson R, Oscarson J, Sundler F (1986) Scand J Gastroenterol 21: Suppl 118, 18-30

21. Hakanson R, Sundler F (1986) Trends Pharmacol Sci 7: 386-387

22. Hall CN, Darkin D, Brimblecombe R, Cook AR, Kirkham JS, Northfield TC (1986) Gut 27: 491-498

23. Hall CN, Kirkham JS, Northfield TC (1987) Gut 28: 216-220

24. Harleman JH, Betton GR, Dormer C, McCrossan M (1987) Scand J Gastroenterol 22: 595-600

25. Hattori T, Halpap B, Gedigk P (1982) Virchows Arch B 38: 283-290

26. Hirth RS (1987) VI International Symposium on Gastrointestinal Toxicologic Pathology, Philadelphia

27. Ito N, Takahashi M, Fukushima S, Shirai T, Tatematsu M (1979) In: Pfeiffer CJ (ed) Gastric cancer. Gerhard Witzstrock, New York, pp277-302

28. Ivankovic S (1979) In: Pfeiffer CJ (Ed) Gastric cancer. Gerhard Witzstrock, New York, pp303-355

29. Kobori O, Oota K (1979) Int J Cancer 23: 536-541

30. Koop H, Arnold R (1987) Internist 28: 8-13

31. Koop H, Schubert B, Schwarting H, Schikierka D, Eissele R, Willemer S, Arnold R (1987) Eur J Clin Invest 17: 111-116

32. Leach SA, Thompson M, Hill M (1987) Carcinogenesis 8: 1907-1912

33. Lewin KJ, Layfield L, Cheng L (1985) Am J Surg Pathol 9: 129-134

34. Martin F, Macleod IB, Sircus W (1970) Gastroenterology 59: 437-444

35. Moody TW, Pert CB, Gazdar AF, Carney DN, Minna JD (1981) Science 214: 1246-1248

36. Morson BC, Sobin LH, Grundmann E, Johansen A, Nagayo T, Serck-Hanssen A (1980) J Clin Path 33: 711-721

37. Nicolson GL (1987) Cancer Res 47: 1473-1487

38. Ohe K, Yagita M, Nagamatsu N, Miura Y, Taoka Y (1987) Gastroenterology 92: 1559

39. Penston JG, Wormsley KG (1986) Med Toxicol 1: 163-168

40. Reed PI, Smith PLR, Haines K, House FR, Walters CL (1981) Lancet 2: 550-

552

41. Reznik-Schuller H (1977) Verh Dtsch Gasellsch Pathol 61: 136-138

42. Rode J, Dhillon AP, Cotton PB Woolf A, O'Riordan JLH (1987) J Clin Pathol 40: 546-551

43. Rode J, Dhillon AP, Papadaki L, Stockbrugger R, Thompson RJ, Moss E, Cotton PB (1986) Gut 27: 789-798

44. Rosko JE, Chang CC (1985) In: Woodhead AD, Shellabarger CJ, Pond V, Hollaender A (eds) Assessment of risk from low-level exposure to radiation and chemicals. Plenum Press, New York, pp261-281

45. Schlag P, Bockler R, Peter M (1982) Scand J Gastroenterol 17: 145-150

46. Schmahl D (1978) Acta Hepato-Gastroenterol 25: 333-334

47. Sharma BK, Santana IA, Wood EC, Walt RP, Pereira M, Noone P, Smith PLR, Walters CL, Pounder RE (1984) Br Med J 289: 717-719

48. Sjoblom SM, Haapiainen R, Mittinen M, Jarvinen H (1987) Acta Chir Scand 153: 37-43

49. Solcia E, Capella C, Sessa F, Rindi G, Cornaggia M, Riva C, Villani L (1986) Digestion 35: Suppl 1, 3-22

50. Stage JG, Bonfils S, Mignon M, Stadil F (1982) Scand J Gastroenterol 17: 401-404

51. Street CS, Cimprich RE, Robertson JL (1984) Scand J Gastroenterol 19: Suppl 101, 109-117

52. Sugimura T, Kawachi T (1973) In: Busch H (Ed) Methods in cancer research, vol VII. Academic Press, New York, pp245-308

53. Sundler F, Hakanson R, Carlsson E, Larsson H, Mattsson H (1986) Digestion 35: Supl 1, 56-69

54. Svendsen JH, Dahl C, Svendsen LB, Christiansen PM (1986) Scand J Gastroenterol 21: 16-20

55. Tahara E, Ito H, Nakagami K, Shimamoto F (1981) Cancer Res Clin Oncol 100: 1-12

56. Tielemans Y, Sundler F, Hakanson R, Willems G (1987) Gastroenterology 92: 1671

57. Weber S, Zuckerman JE, Bostwick DG, Bensch KG, Sikic BI, Raffin TA (1985) J Clin Invest 75: 306-309

58. Wormsley KG (1981) Gut 25: 1416-14232

59. Wormsley KG (1987) Gut 28: 488-505

# GENERAL AETIOLOGY

© *Elsevier Science Publishers B.V. (Biomedical Division)*
*Gastric carcinogenesis. P.I. Reed, M.J. Hill, editors.*

GENETIC INFLUENCES UPON GASTRIC CANCER FREQUENCY

M J S LANGMAN

Department of Medicine, Queen Elizabeth Hospital, Birmingham B15 2TH, UK

INTRODUCTION

Variations in the geographical, social, chronological or familial frequency of gastric cancer may yield important clues to the root causes of disease and help in the formulation of hypotheses suitable for formal testing.

In searching for genetic influences a classical approach has been to examine disease frequency within families of affected probands. However there remain difficulties in deciding whether increases in disease frequency over expectation reflect common inheritance or the influence of the same environmental factors. Evidence for genetic influences may be more firmly established if associations can be shown with specific genetic markers. The possible importance of genetic influences is not diminished by showing that world wide disease patterns are consonant with the variable effects of environmental factors. These may only have their influence upon a population of susceptibles.

FAMILY STUDIES

These have generally shown that disease frequency is increased in family members (1-3) and Table 1 shows data obtained in Denmark.

TABLE 1

DEATHS FROM CANCER OF THE STOMACH IN RELATIVES OF CANCER PATIENTS (10)

|          |          | Deaths   |          |
|----------|----------|----------|----------|
|          | Total No | Observed | Expected |
| Fathers  | 284      | 36       | 13.7     |
| Mothers  | 284      | 25       | 12.6     |
| Brothers | 731      | 33       | 12.6     |
| Sisters  | 684      | 22       | 11.5     |

In rough terms disease frequency was doubled in all close relatives. The fact that this difference was apparent in members of different generations as well as of the same generation is some, if weak, evidence in favour of genetic factor increasing disease liability. It must be remembered, however, that migrant studies suggest that in those who move from an area of high to low disease incidence, there is a delayed fall in disease frequency. This indicates that environmental habits or factors predisposing to disease may be incubated early in life.

Comparisons of outcome on mono and dizygotic twins can give stronger indications of genetic influences upon disease frequency but available data give no clear indications (Table 2).

TABLE 2
TWIN STUDIES IN GASTRIC CANCER - TWINS AFFECTED (5)

|  | Pairs with Cancer | Total Pairs |
|---|---|---|
| Dizygotic | 4 | 58 |
| Monozygotic | 2 | 34 |

On the other hand data obtained in the spouses of patients, if they show no increase in disease frequency over control expectation, can suggest that an excess of disease in blood relatives is due to common inheritance (3). It remains possible, however, that a low disease frequency in spouses could be explained by an impact of critical environmental factors early in life (Table 3).

TABLE 3
CANCER FREQUENCY IN THE SPOUSES OF PATIENTS

| Patients | Total No | Cancer Observed | |
|---|---|---|---|
|  |  | Spouses | Controls |
| Male | 301 | 10 | 8 |
| Female | 249 | 14 | 14 |

RACIAL DIFFERENCES

Although pronounced differences may exist in disease frequency between individuals of different races living in the same area, the variations seem likely to be explained by environmental factors. Thus disease frequency in Japanese migrants to the USA after one generation becomes that of the adopted country.

MARKERS

Individuals of blood group A have been known for forty years to be more susceptible to gastric cancer than those of group O, B or AB (4). This observation arose from linking intellectually a raised frequency of gastric cancer in the North of the United Kingdom with a higher proportion of individuals of blood group O in the general population. In fact, the reverse turned out to be true (5) (Table 4).

TABLE 4

PROPORTIONS OF INDIVIDUALS OF BLOOD GROUP A IN SELECTED SERIES (8)

| | Cases | | Controls | |
|---|---|---|---|---|
| | No | % | No | % |
| Europe | | | | |
| London | 1340 | 46.0 | 1340 | 42.3 |
| Paris | 1457 | 48.0 | 207588 | 44.0 |
| Milan | 678 | 48.2 | 2346 | 41.8 |
| Copenhagen | 854 | 48.4 | 6299 | 44.0 |
| Japan | | | | |
| Sendai | 1671 | 40.1 | 21199 | 36.7 |
| Sapporo | 1565 | 42.2 | 1937 | 37.3 |
| USA | | | | |
| Connecticut | 892 | 45.0 | 30601 | 40.3 |

Disease tends to be about twenty percent more common in individuals of group A, and the reasons are unclear. Genetically, any individual has the ability to produce blood group substances of the ABO (H) type in water soluble form or not to do so, and to produce Lewis group substances instead, the distinction being by the sugar moiety of the molecules. The excess of individuals of group A is not associated with any change in the properties of secretory or non-secretory status, suggesting that simple expression of blood group substances in the mucous secretons is irrelevant.

The same excess of blood group A is detectable in pernicious anaemia (6) and this is again of about twenty percent. However, individuals with pernicious anaemia who develop gastric cancer do not seem to be peculiarly likely to be of group A nor have any other obvious differences been noted from ordinary gastric cancer (3).

In attempting to understand or refine the ABO blood group association with gastric cancer two different approaches can be made. Firstly, attempts can be made to relate findings to other blood group associations affecting physiological or biochemical function. Secondly, associations might be sought with particular sets of cancer patients.

FUNCTIONAL ASSOCIATIONS

## Secretion

No coherent set of data exists to allow the ABO Blood group association to be related to acid output. However, there is an association with a secretion of protein but not immunoglobulin levels in (salivary) secretion (6,11). The difference in levels between individuals of the ABO Blood groups is large, but there is no obvious link with liability to gastric cancer.

## Alkaline Phosphatase Polymorphism

Individuals of blood groups O and B, are particularly likely to release intestinal alkaline phosphatase into their circulation but individuals of group A are less likely to do so (7). Two additional pieces of information suggest, however, that this polymorphism is irrelevant. Firstly, the ability to release alkaline phosphatase is governed overridingly by secretor status and there is no evidence that this influences disease liability. Secondly, gastric cancer of intestinal type may be that which is less likely to be associated with the blood groups.

## Cancer Subsite

Examination of the ABO blood groups in individuals with cancer at specific subsites has shown no consistent trend, some suggesting that blood group A is particularly associated with cancer of the body of the stomach, and others the reverse.

## Histological Type

Data from Colombia and Hawaii suggest that group A may be particularly associated with the diffuse type of disease (Table 5).

TABLE 5

PROPORTIONS OF INDIVIDUALS OF GROUP A ACCORDING TO HISTOLOGICAL SUBTYPE OF CANCER (4)

| | % Group A | | |
| | General Population | Diffuse Cancer | Intestinal Cancer |
|---|---|---|---|
| Colombia | 18 | 35 | 22 |
| Japanese | 38 | 49 | 39 |

| Relative risk | Diffuse type | Colombia | 2.45:1 |
|---|---|---|---|
| | | Japanese | 1.57:1 |
| | Intestinal type | Colombia | 1.28:1 |
| | | Japanese | 1.04:1 |

Geographical Pathology

Findings generally hold good in all areas, irespective of whether disease frequency is low or high.

EVIDENCE OF DIVERSITY IN DISEASE

Gastric cancer has generally been considered as a homogeneous entity. However, division into two histological subtypes, intestinal and diffuse, has suggested that the main chronological changes in disease frequency occur because of alterations in the incidence of the intestinal type of disease. Searches for genetic factors may, therefore, be more effective if disease is considered in these separate categories.

In addition, it seems that although general disease frequency may be falling, the overall change may conceal variations by subsite.

Table 6 shows the overall fall in disease incidence in men in the West Midlands Region of England.

TABLE 6

GASTRIC CANCER, AGE SPECIFIC INCIDENCE PER 100,000 PER YEAR. WEST MIDLANDS, UK MEN

| Age | 1960-62 | 68-72 | 79-82 |
|-----|---------|-------|-------|
| 40- | 18.6 | 7.6 | 6.2 |
| 50- | 61.6 | 31.3 | 26.0 |
| 60- | 163.9 | 100.6 | 76.4 |

A roughly equivalent trend is also discernible in women. Division of the available cases according to sex and time (Table 7) suggests an increasing preponderance of men despite a general tendency in the population at large for the proportion of women to be greater in the elderly, those most at risk of gastric cancer.

Further subdivision by tumour site in the stomach indicates a rising number of tumours in the cardia, mainly in men, but lesser change in the amount of pyloric disease. The reasons for all these changes are obscure but they underline the need to consider gastric cancer as a heterogenous entity.

TABLE 7

NUMBER OF TUMOURS BY SITE W MIDLANDS, UK

|  | 1957-61 | 1967-71 | 1977-81 |
|---|---|---|---|
| Cardia | 281 | 563 | 923 |
| Pylorus | 1143 | 1338 | 1436 |
| All other | 4138 | 4609 | 3948 |

Male to female ratio

|  | 1957-61 | 1967-71 | 1977-81 |
|---|---|---|---|
| Cardia |  |  |  |
| M | 205 | 421 | 709 |
| F | 76 | 142 | 214 |
| Ratio | 0.37 | 0.34 | 0.34 |

FUTURE PROSPECTS

The advent of molecular biological techniques should transform our understanding of genetic influences on disease frequency. One indication of what may be in store is recent evidence that genetic factors on chromosome 5 have important influences upon liability to colonic cancer (9).

REFERENCES

1.  A collective series from a number of centres (1956) ii:723-4

2.  Aird I, Bentall HH, Roberts JAF (1953) Brit Med J i:799-801

3.  Callender S, Langman MJS, MacLeod IN, Mosbech J, Nielsen RK (1971) Gut 12:465-467

4.  Correa P, Haenszel W (1982) In: Correa P, Haenszel W (eds) Epidemiology of cancer of the digestive tract. Martirins Nijhoff, The Hague

5.  Hauge M, Harvald B (1961) Acta Genet (Basel) 11:372-378

6.  Hope RM, Mayo O, Boettcher B (1968) Vox Sang (Basel) 15:70-74

7.  Langman MJS, Leuthold E, Robson EB, Harris J, Luffman JE, Harris H (1966) Nature 212:41-43

8.  McConnell RB (1966) The Genetics of Gastrointestinal Disorders. Oxford University Press, London

9.  Solomon E, Voss R, Hall V, Bodmer WF, Joss JR, Jeffreys AJ, Lucibello FC, Patel I, Rider SH (1987) 328:616-619

10. Videback A, Mosbech J (1954) Acta Med Scand 1149:137-159

11. Waissbluth JG, Langman MJS (1971) Gut: 646-649

12. Woolf CM (1961) Cancer 14:199-200

© Elsevier Science Publishers B.V. (Biomedical Division)
Gastric carcinogenesis. P.I. Reed, M.J. Hill, editors.

DIETARY FACTORS IN THE AETIOLOGY OF GASTRIC CANCER

PATRICIA A JUDD

Department of Food and Nutritional Sciences, Kings College London (KQG), Campden Hill Road, London W8 7AH

INTRODUCTION

Although the incidence of gastric carcinoma has been decreasing throughout the world during the last 30 years, it is still possibly one of the most common cancers worldwide, particularly in men. (52). It seems reasonable, as the stomach is an organ which has prolonged contact with foods, that dietary factors would be involved in the aetiology of the disease. In addition, a variety of carcinogens and co-carcinogens are known to be present in the human diet (59) although it has not yet been possible to identify specific compounds involved in gastric cancer with any certainty.

The logical idea that differences in dietary habits are involved in the fall in incidence has been pursued energeticaly for the last 25 years or so. However, in western countries, where the decline in incidence was first observed, there have been many changes in lifestyle as well as in dietary habits which make the aetiology difficult to establish. Two developments have given new impetus to investigations. Firstly, the classification of GC into two subgroups, the so-called intestinal and diffuse types of Lauren in 1965 (40) allowed the re-examination of geographical epidemiology. It was thus demonstrated that variations in prevalence of the disease between countries are mainly due to differences in prevalence of the intestinal type - ie that which appears to be associated wtih environmental factors (12). Secondly an hypothesis put forward by Correa et al (13) and since expanded (11) outlined a possible mechanism for the development of the intestinal type of gastric carcinoma which allowed direct research into the environmental causes, enabling the disorder to be seen as developing in a series of stages. This gives the possibility of investigating causative factors early in the natural history, before the disease has resulted in changes in diet or lifestyle. It has also provided a mechanism by which some of the results of epidemiological studies can be explained and enabled more recent workers to refine their questioning.

It is postulated that the first step in development of gastric cancer involves chronic superficial gastritis, a condition which is completely reversible if the causative factors can be identified and removed. The next stage in progression is the development of chronic atrophic gastritis, with loss of parietal cell mass, eventually resulting in hypochlorhydria. This allows bacterial overgrowth in the stomach. Some bacteria contain nitrate reductases which transform dietary nitrates to nitrite, an extremely active molecule which may combine with many possible substrates eg secondary amines or amides in foods and drugs and possibly bile acids to form mutagenic N-nitroso compounds (54). The N-nitroso compounds may be involved in increasingly severe dysplasia and eventually carcinoma; certainly such compounds have been shown to be carcinogenic in animals (44).

There are various points in the process postulated above where dietary factors may come into play. As well as acting as initiating or promoting factors it is possible that some dietary components are protective eg vitamins C, and E (together with Selenium), vitamin A or carotenoids. The following sections will outline the problems which arise in the determination of dietary factors in gastric cancer; foods and nutrients which have been suggested to be important and possible mechanisms for their effects.

## METHODOLOGY OF DIETARY STUDIES

Measuring food and nutrient intakes has often been regarded as relatively easy - the tools required are simple and with the advent of computerised dietary data banks the once combersome conversion of foods into nutrient content has been speeded up immensely. However, it is in fact notoriously difficult to obtain accurate information about individuals diets and a recent review (5) has suggested that many of the methods which have been used in cancer epidemiology have not been well validated and may not be capable of giving the results required ie the classification of individuals into extremes of population distributtion.

Several reviews evaluating methods used to assess dietary intake have been published (3,5,7,41). In most cases the methods described are intended to measure current food consumption and all have their drawbacks. Table 1 shows the possible sources of error when using different methods.

The most common method against which many others are validated is the precise weighing method where subjects are asked to weigh all food and drink eaten over a period of time and record this on paper or possibly on audio tape. Variations on this include using household measures instead of weights, with the attendant problem of how to assign correct weights to foods. The food consumption data are then converted into nutrients using standard food composition data for the particular country. In most countries this data is limited to basic foods and dishes and cannot acocunt for the huge range of foods available today.

Cancer, including gastric cancer, develop over a period of years, possibly decades, and dietary factors may be involved at the initiation or promotion stages or in both. A further problem in case control studies is that it is never known whether the findings are a cause or consequence of the disease studied. This is particularly so in diseases where symptoms may cause changes in eating habits, either voluntarily or on medical advice. Patients with gastric cancer are such a group and it is therefore desirable to try to ascertain eating habits before symptoms developed.

TABLE 1

SOURCES OF ERROR IN DIETARY SURVEYS (ADAPTED FROM BINGHAM, REF 5)

| Source of Error | Weighed Records | Records with Estimated Weights | 24hr Recall | Diet History and Questionnaires |
|---|---|---|---|---|
| Sampling bias | + | + | + | + |
| Response bias | +/- | +/- | +/- | +/- |
| Food tables | + | + | + | + |
| Coding errors | + | + | + | + |
| Wrong food weight | - | + | + | + |
| Reporting error | - | - | + | + |
| Variation with time | + | + | + | - |
| Wrong frequency of consumption | - | - | - | + |
| Change in diet | +/- | +/- | - | - |

In this situation measuring current intake is obviously inappropriate and there is, instead, a need for reliable and accurate measures of assessing past dietary intake. Information is required not only about nutrient intakes but also about food consumption patterns eg frequency of use of dairy products, vegetables or meat products and it is also desirable to collect information about cooking methods as carcinogenic compounds may form during frying or grilling. (62). Further information may also be required about non-nutritive factors such as nitrates, nitrites or food additives.

Some form of recall method would therefore seem to be more appropriate for use in epidemiology. The simplest of these is the 24 hour recall where people are asked by a trained interviewer to recall all foods and drinks taken during the previous 24 hours. This has been put forward as a valid method for assessing the mean intakes of large groups of people (10) although Bingham questions this assumption and points out that extensive validation is essential in each particular study (5). It is not suitable for studies of diet and cancer, where it is the habitual diet of individuals or small groups of people which is of interest.

Many workers have used dietary histories for looking at past food intake. The dietary history as originally described by Burke (8) consisted of three parts: a 24 hour recall, questions about frequency of consumption of a list of around 100 foods and a three day record of foods eaten. The dietary history aims to determine the food pattern of an individual over a defined period of time from about one month to one year. A dietitian or specially-trained nutritionist asks the respondant about consumption of different foods or dishes over the specified time. Food models or photographs may be used to determine portion sizes or standard portions may be used and there are cross-checks within the questioning to enable as accurate a picture as possible to be built up. Diet history methods are known to give higher estimates of nutrient intakes than food records but have been said to have good reproducibility by some workers (18,51). However Bingham again questions this, suggesting that insufficient comparisons have been made between this method and food records.

The dietary history method is time consuming (at least 90 minutes/subject) and expensive since trained personnel are needed and so is not suitable for large population studies. It is often used in case-control studies and many modifications of the original method have been devised so it is essential that a full description of methodology be given in publications. This should include details of the number of items in the questionnaire, food frequency categories and method of estimating portion size as well as information on validity and reliability (53).

There is a continuing search for less time-consuming and cheaper retrospective methods. Self administered dietary history questionnaires have been developed and provided they are properly validated and tested for reliability can save time and money. Such a questionnaire has been used in the Finnish cancer prevention trial (53). The use of food frequency questionnaires is another simplification of the dietary history method. These attempts to measure habitual food patterns by asking about the use of a limited number of foods which have been included in order to test a particular hypothesis. This method has been used quite frequently in studies on gastrointestinal cancers and has been found to have reasonably good validity and good reproducibility when comparing the frequency or group mean intakes of foods or food groups (2,27,47,57). However, it is less straight-forward when looking at nutrient intakes as it is not always easy to be sure that the foods selected are true index foods and validity and reliability data has rarely been reported for such questionnaires (53). Portion size estimations are sometimes included but some workers feel that this does not necessarily improve the quality of the results (Byers, personal communication).

Measures of Food Intake in the Distant Past

Given the difficulty that many people experience in remembering recent food intake, measurement of diet from years earlier seems an unlikely proposition and it is considered by some to be virtually impossible (5). However various attempts have been made to validate such methods by comparing diet history or food frequency questionnaires with data collected some years ago. Several authors have concluded that the retrospective diet is overinfluenced by current diet (21,35) although in one study usual frequency of intake of foods reported 20 years previously was in better agreement with the originally reported data than current diet (9). If the patient has recently changed their diet because of their disease the influence of current diet is likely to be even more of a problem. A further complication in the UK and possibly other countries at present is the great deal of space given in the popular media to ideas about nutrition and diet which may also influence the respondants, whether cases or controls.

It must therefore be apparent that identifying foods or nutrients involved in the aetiology of gastric cancer is no easy task. It is possible that some of the risk factors which have surfaced in epidemiological studies may be quite spurious but nevertheless connections can be seen between widely differing communities with respect to dietary factors which may be important clues to aetiology.

## FOODS AND NUTRIENTS POSITIVELY OR NEGATIVELY ASSOCIATED WITH GC

Recent reviews have summarised the evidence for involvement of dietary factors in gastric carcinogenesis (6,22,44) and Table 2 shows the foods and food components which have been positively or negatively associated with GC risk. In early studies no clear picture emerged and the dietary factors appeared to be different from country to country. For example smoked fish was associated with high risk in Iceland (19) and for immigrants of Norweigan origin in Minnesota (6) but in Japan fish is not usually smoked and the association is therefore not found. However, fish either fresh, dried or salted has been shown to be a risk factor in studies of Japanese in Japan and Hawaii (25,31). Fava beans appear to be associated with increased risk in Columbia (39), soup in Norway (6), beef in Japan (48) and chocolate in Canada (55), Japan and elsewhere (25,45).

As informtion accumulated, however it became possible to identify links between the dietary factors and there now seems to be a concensus as to the type of diet characteristic of populations with gastric carcinoma. Correa (15) has summarised the general characteristics of such diets (see Table 3).

TABLE 2

FOOD AND COMPONENTS OF FOODS WHICH HAVE BEEN SUGGESTED TO BE ASSOCIATED WITH HIGH OR LOW RISK OF GC

| High Risk | Low Risk |
|---|---|
| Added salt | High fat |
| Salted foods eg fish, bacon | Milk |
| Smoked foods eg meat, fish | High intake of fresh |
| Fish (fresh, dried, salted) | fruits and vegetables |
| Animal and cooked fats | Vitamin C |
| Fried foods | Vitamin E, selenium |
| Pickles (including pickled vegetables) | |
| Rice (as stabple food) and rice cakes | |
| Potatoes | |
| Cooked cereals | |
| Canned fruit: fresh fruit | |
| Fava beans | |
| Alcohol | |
| Cabbage | |
| Beef | |
| Chocolate | |
| Hot tea | |
| Milk | |

TABLE 3

CHARACTERISTICS OF THE DIETS OF POPULATIONS AT HIGH RISK OF GC

1. Low intake of animal fats and protein
2. High intakes of starches and carbohydrates, mainly from grains and starchy roots
3. High salt intakes
4. High dietary nitrate intakes (from water or foodstuffs)
5. Low intakes of fresh fruits
6. Low intake of raw vegetables and salads

General Dietary Patterns

In many countries these dietary patterns are characteristic of sections of the population with low economic status (34,64) and in some cases particular occupations, such as manual work in coal mines and oil refineries are associated with high incidence of the disease (17,58) although it has been suggested that low socioeconomic status is important rather than occupation per se. It is quite possible that some of the reduction in incidence is associated with changes in diet and lifestyle which accompany increased socioeconomic status, for example this may result in increased intake of animal proteins or fruits and vegetables as demonstrated in a recent study from Poland (34) or there may be decreased intake of smoked or salted foods as access to refrigeration improves. Other beneficial effects of cold storage are said to be due to its mould-inhibiting properties and to the inhibition of nitrite formation in preserved foods (61).

Salt and Salted Foods

As can be seen from Table 1, salted foods of various types eg bacon (28,42) fish, (6,25,26,39) or just salted foods generally (26,30,56) appeared to be associated with higher risks. Pickled foods and sauces are often also high in salt and these too appear to more commonly eaten by high risk groups (25,31,39,48). Geboers and coworkers (22) have looked at the evidence for the role of salt in gastric carcinogenesis in a different way, based on the early observations by Joossens that both within and between countries there is a strong association between mortality from stroke and GC. It is virtually impossible to measure dietary salt intakes in free-living populations but significant positive correlations between salt as measured by 24 hour urinary sodium and both GC and stroke have been shown (36). A short report from a study looking at Na excretion in the urine of teenage girls from 3 countries with differing GC incidences also supports the salt hypothesis; levels of Na excretion were lowest in the USA, intermediate in Chile and highest in Japan, in parallel with GC incidence (4). Some workers have also included questions about addition of salt to foods as a rough guide to salt intake and suggest that there are more habitual salt users in cases that in control groups (16) or that people who classify themselves as 'heavy users' of salt had a higher relative risk (20). The role of salt is discussed in greater detail elsewhere in this volume by Joossens and Kestoloot.

Dietary Nitrate, Nitrite and N-nitroso Compounds

Nitrates are present in foods either because they are added during preservation of meats or fish or because foods are grown on soils naturally high in nitrate or enriched by extensive use of nitrate fertilisers. The idea that nitrate in foods is important is therefore supported by some of the data from Table 1. For example bacon (28,42) and the cured meats (16) will be high in nitrates as may grains in some situations (26) and vegetables (including fava beans). However raw vegetables and fruits are usually found to be associated with lower risks and it has been suggested that it is not the amount of nitrate as such which is important but the amount which can be converted to nitrite in the stomach (16). Thus in areas where nitrate is eaten in raw salad, fresh green leafy vegetables or fresh fruit protective factors may be present which prevent the reduction of nitrate to nitrite.

Nitrites may be present in bacon and cured meat but in recent years changes in food processing have reduced the amounts markedly. Preformed N-nitroso compounds may also be found in some foodstuffs such as cured meats, fish and beers (54).

Low Intakes of Fresh Fruits and Vegetables

As mentioned above, high intakes of raw vegetables (16,24,25) fresh fruits and vegetables (6,15,45) lettuce (6,23,24) or green/yellow vegetables (30) have been negatively associated with GC risk. In other studies vitamin C has been identified as a protective factor (16,39,55). Studies have shown that Vitamin C does reduced intragastric nitrosation (33,43) and this may therefore be important. However, other dietary components present in fruits and vegetables, such as tannins and polyphenols, (43) vitamin E (43,50) or carotenoids (6,16) may also be protective because of their role as antioxidants.

Individual 'High Risk' Foods or Protective Factors

There are some foods or nutrients which cannot be categorised in general terms but which nevertheless have emerged as risk factors. Fish has been isolated in several studies in countries here it is an important part of the diet (22). It has been shown in animal studies that certain types of fish yield produts with direct mutagenic activity on reaction with nitrite at pH 3 and that the reaction is inhibited by vitamin C (62). Fava beans also yield potentially mutagenic compounds (46,65).

Milk is a food which has been associated with both high (20) and low risk (29). It has been suggested, however, that the positive association may be due to a higher consumption of milk in patients who use it to relieve gastric discomfort (20,45). Recently, Nelson and coworders observed a high consumption of sterilised milk in a community with high incidence of gastric cancer and suggested that the prolonged heat treatment might destroy protective factors found in milk. Alternatively it may be that consumption of this type of milk is just a marker for a generally poor diet (49).

Alcohol is known to be a gastric irritant and it has been implicated as a risk factor for gastric cancer in several studies (16,30,32,64). Other workers have not found alcohol to be a significant risk factor (1,24).

Fig. 1. A model for gastric carcinogenesis

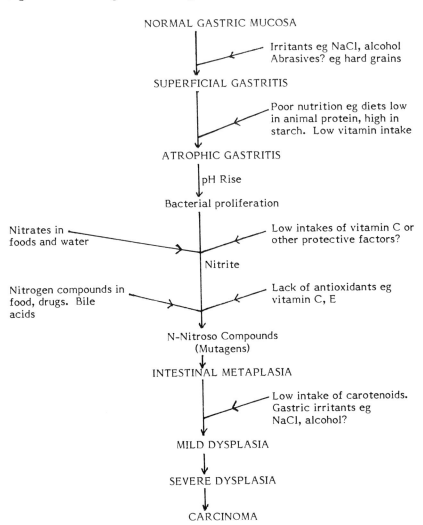

NORMAL GASTRIC MUCOSA

Irritants eg NaCl, alcohol
Abrasives? eg hard grains

SUPERFICIAL GASTRITIS

Poor nutrition eg diets low
in animal protein, high in
starch. Low vitamin intake

ATROPHIC GASTRITIS

pH Rise

Bacterial proliferation

Nitrates in foods and water    Low intakes of vitamin C or other protective factors?

Nitrite

Nitrogen compounds in food, drugs. Bile acids    Lack of antioxidants eg vitamin C, E

N-Nitroso Compounds
(Mutagens)

INTESTINAL METAPLASIA

Low intake of carotenoids.
Gastric irritants eg
NaCl, alcohol?

MILD DYSPLASIA

SEVERE DYSPLASIA

CARCINOMA

(Adapted from Correa 1984)

## The 'Correa Model' of Development of GC and Mechanisms whereby Diet May Affect It

Fig 1 presents in diagrammatic form a possible model for the development of gastric cancer (adapted from Correa, 14). It is possible to explain some of the association betwen diet and gastric cancer using this model and it is now being used as a basis of studies looking at diet at earlier stages in the development of the disease. Some of the factors associated with GC also appear to hold true in patients with chronic atrophic gastritis (20) and this is discussed in greater detail elsewhere in this volume.

Other hypotheses for the role of diet in GC do exist but have perhaps not been submitted to as much investigation as that of Correa et al (13). It has been suggested for example that high intakes of polyunsaturated fats may yield lipid peroxides or that high intakes of dietary linoleic acid may result in production of 'free radicals' either of which might participate in carcinogenesis (38,63). Lipid-phase antioxidants such as vitamin E may inhibit these processes and other minor food components may suppress neoplasm formation in cells previously exposed to carcinogens (60). Risch (55) reported that only beta-carotene out of several minor constituents including retinoids, seeds and legumes (a source of protease inhibitors) and crucifereous vegetables showed up as a possible protective factor.

## CONCLUSIONS

Given that methods of measuring diet in the distant past are fraught with problems and that it may have changed due to symptoms of disease, the identificaton of atrophic gastritis as a precursor lesion should prove useful. At this stage patients symptoms may not be affecting dietary habits and it is possible that the period over which they are asked to remember their diet is less distant. It may therefore be possible to identify factors involved in the early stages of the disease. Perhaps more useful though is the opportunity to carry out a prospective study on such patients using the best possible measures of current diet and repeating this at intervals. It may then be possible to identify the dietary charcateristics which prevent the continued development of the disease.

## REFERENCES

1.    Acheson ED and Doll R (1964) Gut 5:126-545

2.    Axelson JM, Csernus MM (1983) J Am Diet Assoc 83:152-155

3.    Bazarre TL and Myers MP (1980) Nutr Cancer 1:22-45

4.    Bernstein L and Henderson BE (1985) J Canc Res Clin Oncol 110 (2):184

5.    Bingham S (1987) Nutrition Abstracts and Reviews. (Series A) 57:705-742

6.    Bjelke E (1974) Scand J Gastroenterol 9 (Supple 31):1-253

7.   Block G (1982) Am J epidemiol 115:492-505

8.   Burke BS (1947) J Am Diet Assoc 23:1041-1046

9.   Byers TE, Rosenthal RI, Marshall JR, Rzepka TF, Cummings KM, Graham S (1983) Nutrition and Cancer 5:69-77

10.  Cole T and Black AE (1983) In The dietary assessment of populations. MRC Environmental Epidemiology Unit Report. Southampton General Hospital, Southampton, England

11.  Correa P (1983) Cancer Surveys 2:437-450

12.  Correa P, Susano N, Stemmerman GN et al (1973) J Natl Cancer Inst 51:1449-1459

13.  Correa P, Haenszel W, Cuello C, Archer M and Tannenbaum S (1975) Lancet 2:58-60

14.  Correa P (1984) Scand J Gastroenterol 19 suppl 104:131-136

15.  Correa (1985) Seminars in Oncology, 12:2-10

16.  Correa P, Fontham E, Pickle LW, Chen V, Lin Y and Haenszel W (1985) JNCI 75(4):645-654

17.  Davies JM (1980) Br J Cancer 41:438-455

18.  Dawber TR, Pearson G, Anderson P, Mann GV, Kannel WB, Swartleff D, McNamara P (1962) Am J Clin Nutr 11:226-234

19.  Dungal N (1961) JAMA 178:789-798

20.  Fontham E, Zavala D, Correa P, Rodriguez E, Hunter F, Haenszel, W and Tannenbaum SR 91986) JNCI 76:621-627

21.  Garland B, Ibrahim M, Grimson R (1982) Am J Epidemiology 116:577 (abstract)

22.  Geboers J, Joossens JV and Kesteloot H (1985) In Joossens JV, Hill MJ and Geboers J (eds) Diet and human carcinogenesis. Excerta Medica, Amsterdam-New York-Oxford p81-95

23.  Graham S, Lillienfield AM, Tidings JE (1967) Cancer 20:2224-2234

24.  Graham S, Schotz W, Martino P (1972) Cancer 30:927-938

25.  Haenszel W, Kurihara M, Segi M, Lee RK (1972) J Natl Cancer Inst 49:969-988

26.  Haenszel W, Kurihara M, Locke FB, Shimuzu K, Segi M (1976) J Natl Cancer Inst 56:265-278

27.  Hankin JH, Rhoads GG, glober GA (1975) Am J Clin Nutr 28:1055-1061

28.  Higginson J (1966) J Natl, Cancer Inst 37:527-545

29.  Hirayama T (1967) Unio Intern Contre Cancrum Monogr 10:37-48

30.  Hirayama T (1971) GANN Monogr Cancer Res 11:3-19

31.  Hirayama T (1975) Cancer Research 35:3460-3463

32.  Hoey J, Montevernay C, Lambert R Am J epidemiol 113:668-674

33.  Iqbal ZM, epstein SS, Krull IS, Goff U, Mills K, Fine DH (1980) In Walker EA, Griciute L, Castegnaro M, Borszsonyi M, Davies W eds. N-nitroso compounds. Analysis, formation and occurrence. IARC Scientific Publ 1980 31:169-182

34.  Jedrychowski WA, Popiels T 91986) Neoplasma 33:97-106

35.  Jenson OM, Wahrendorf J, Rosenquist A, Geser A 91984) Am J epidemiol 120:281-290

36. Joossens JV, Geboers J (1981) Nutr Cancer 2:250-261

37. Joossens JV, Geboers J (1983) In Sherlock P, Morson BC, Barbara L, Veronesi U. (eds) Precancerous lesions of the Gastrointestinal tract. New York; Raven press pp97-113

38. King MM, McCay PB (1983) Cancer Res (suppl) 43:2485-2490s

39. Kolonel LN, Nomura AMY, Hirohata T, Hankin JH, Hinds MW (1981) Am J Clin Nutr 34: 2478-2485

40. Lauren P (1965) Acta Pathologica et Microbiologica Scandinavica 64:31-49

41. Marr J (1971) Individual dietary surveys: purposes and methods. World Review of Nutrition and Dietetics 13:105-164

42. Meinsma L (1964) voeding 25:357-365

43. Mirvish SS (1981) In Burchenal JH, Oettgen HF eds Cancer 1980: Achievements, challenges, prospects for the 1980's. New York: Grune, 1981:557-587

44. Mirvish SS (1983) J Natl Cancer Inst 71(3):631-647

45. Modan B, Lubin F, Barell V et al (1974) Cancer 34:2087-2092

46. Montes G, Cuello C, Correa P et al (1984) Nutr Cancer 6:191-195

47. Mullen B, Krantzler NJ, Grivetti LE (1984) Am J clin Nutr 39:136-142

48. Nagai M, Hashimoto T, Yanagwa H (1982) Nutr Cancer 3:257-268

49. Nelson M (1983) Food production and sales. In the dietary assessment of popultions. MRC epidemiology unit report. Southampton General Hospital, Southampton, England

50. Newmark HL, Mergens WJ (1981) Lipkin M, eds Inhibition of tumor induction and development. New York Plenum 1981:127-168

51. Nomura A, Hankin RH, Rhoads GG (1976) Am J Clin Nutr 29:1432-1436

52. Parkin DM, Stjernsward J and Muir CS (1984) Bull or World Health Organisation 62:163-182

53. Pietinen P (1985) In Diet and Human Carcinogenesis eds Joossens JV, Hill MJ and Geboers J. Excerpta Medica Amsterdam-New York-London

54. Reed PI (1985) Human carcinogenesis eds Joossens JV, Hill MJ and Geboers J. Excerpta Medica Amsterdam-New York-London

55. Risch HA, Jain M, Won Choi N, Fodor G, Pfeiffer C, Howe GR, Harrison L, Craib KJP, Miller AB (1985) Am J epidemiol 122(6):947-959

56. Sato T, Fukuyama T, Suzuki T (1959) Bull Inst Publ Health (Japan) 8:187-198

57. Stefanik PA, Trulson MF (1962) Am J Clin Nutr 11:335-343

58. Thomas TL, Waxweiler RJ, Moure-Eraso R, ItaYa S, Fraumeni JF Jnr (1982) J Occup Med 24:131-141

59. Thompson M (1984) Scand J Gastroenterol 19, (Supp 104):77-89

60. Wattenberg LW (1983) Cancer Res (Suppl) 43:2448-2453S

61. Weisberger JH and Raineri R (1975) Cancer Res 35:3469-3474

62. Weisberger JH, Horn CL (1984) Scand J Gastroenterol (supp) 104:15-26

63. Witting LA (1975) Am J Clin Nutr 27:952-959

64. Wynder EL, Kmet K, dungal N, Segi M (1963) Cancer 16:1461-1496

65. Yang D, Tannenbaum SR, Buchi G et al (1984) Carcinogenesis 5:1219-1224

© *Elsevier Science Publishers B.V. (Biomedical Division)*
*Gastric carcinogenesis. P.I. Reed, M.J. Hill, editors.*

# MICRONUTRIENTS AND TRACE ELEMENTS IN CANCER PREVENTION

A T DIPLOCK

Division of Biochemistry, United Medical and Dental Schools, (Universityy of London), Guy's Hospital, London SE1 9RT, UK

## INTRODUCTION

The rapid recent increase in knowledge of the importance of free radical events in biology has caused an explosive growth in speculation about the involvement of free radicals in human disease. Of particular importance are the various free radical and other metabolites of dioxygen, which may arise as normal adjuncts to the process of respiration. The containment of these, and the prevention of their potential detrimental effect on cellular macromolecules, depends ultimately on a number of trace elements and other micronutrients, the absence from, or low supply of which in, the diet may have detrimental consequences in terms of human health. Among the diseases that may involve free radical attack on sensitive micromolecules in their aetiology is cancer in some, or even all, of its multiple forms. In this short article a general review will be given of the biochemical processes that are believed to cause free-radical damage, of their containment by micronutrients or micronutrient-derived enzyme systems, and of the evidence that begins to suggest that increasing intake of these micronutrients may afford protection against carcinogenesis.

## FREE RADICAL FORMATION AND CONTAINMENT

The reduction of molecular dioxygen to water involves the sequential addition of four electrons to the dioxygen molecule. During this process molecular species are formed that have the potential for serious damage to living cells if their reactivity is not kept in check; fortunately under normal nutritional circumstances damage is contained. The sequence of oxygen reduction may be summarised as follows.

$$O_2 \xrightarrow{\quad e \quad} O_2^{\cdot -} \quad \text{(Superoxide anion radical)}$$

$$O_2^{\cdot -} \xrightarrow{\quad e \quad} O_2^{--} \quad \text{(Peroxyl anion)}$$

$$O_2^{--} \xrightarrow{\quad 2H^+ \quad} H_2O_2 \quad \text{(Hydrogen peroxide)}$$

$$H_2O_2 \xrightarrow{\quad H^+,e \quad} (H^+OH^-) + OH^{\cdot} \quad \text{(Hydroxyl radical)}$$

$$OH^{\cdot} \xrightarrow{\quad H^+,e \quad} (H^+OH^-)$$

Overall: $O_2 + 4H^+ \xrightarrow{\quad 4e \quad} 2H_2O$

The potentially damaging molecular species are $O_2^{\cdot-}, O_2^{--}$ (or $H_2O_2$) and, of particular potential cytotoxicity, the hydroxyl radical $OH^{\cdot}$. Under normal circumstances, containment of this risk depends upon a highly sophisticated array of protective mechanisms that can be envisaged as providing three different levels of protection. In the first line of defence, the existence of the superoxide anion radical $O_2^{\cdot-}$, and of hydrogen peroxide, is very transient because they are removed under the catalytic influence of three enzyme systems. The superoxide dismutases (SODS) are responsible for the following reaction:

$$2O_2^{\cdot-} \xrightarrow{\hspace{2cm}} O_2 \qquad\qquad +H_2O$$

Two such enzymes are known to exist in mammalian cells depending on their intracellular localisation: in mitochondria there is a manganese-dependent enzyme which is of entirely different protein structure to the cytosolic enzyme which contains Cu and Zn. The catalytic activity of these enzymes depends upon an adequate nutritional supply of all these three metals, so that dietary deficiency of any or all of them may have disastrous consequences in terms of the cytotoxicity of the superoxide anion radical. The containment of proliferation of $H_2O_2$ depends upon two enzymes; catalase, which catalyses the following reaction:

$$2H_2O_2 \xrightarrow{\text{Catalase}} 2H_2O + O_2$$

and glutathione peroxidase (GSHpx), which catalyses the following:

$$H_2O_2 + 2GSH \xrightarrow{\hspace{1cm}\text{GSHpx}\hspace{1cm}} 2H_2O + GSSG$$

The intracellular localisation of glutathione peroxidase within the cytosol and within the mitochondrial compartment ensures protection in both locations. The enzyme is a selenium-containing protein and the catalytic activity of the enzyme depends upon the presence of four atoms of selenium per mole of enzyme protein. Thus, nutritional inadequacy of selenium may lead to accummulation of hydrogen peroxide within cells which may have serious biological consequences. In the event that marginal dietary inadequacies occur of any or all of the trace elements Mn, Cu, Zn and Se, generation of substantial quantities of the $OH^{\cdot}$ radical may occur, due to the following reaction:

$$O_2^{\cdot-} + H_2O_2 \xrightarrow{\hspace{2cm}} OH^{\cdot} + OH^- + O_2$$

Although this reaction is of limited significance without catalysis at neutral pH, it may be catalysed by the very small amounts of free iron that are to be found in mammalian cells thus:

$$O_2^{\cdot-} \quad \xrightarrow{\phantom{aa}Fe^{3+}\phantom{aa}} \quad O_2 + Fe^{2+}$$

$$H_2O_2 \quad \xrightarrow{\phantom{aa}Fe^{2+}\phantom{aa}} \quad OH^- + OH^{\cdot} + Fe^{3+}$$

Generation of OH$^{\cdot}$ in this way is thought to be of major significance in the aetiology and pathogenesis of a number of disease processes, and containment of the primary metabolites $O_2^{\cdot-}$ and $H_2O_2$ is thus a matter of the utmost importance.

The question of the targets for attack by activated oxygen species requires careful consideration. In the present context of possible mutagenic and carcinogenic effects of free radicals, the fact of substantial evidence of damage to DNA by oxygen radicals provides the most clear link between the underlying biochemistry and the carcinogenic process, and in this the highly reactive OH$^{\cdot}$ radical is potentially the most damaging because of its ability to react rapidly with any DNA molecule with which it comes into contact. However, the significance of attack by oxygen radicals on other macromolecules must not be overlooked. Proteins, including intracellular enzymes, are also likely targets, although study of this area has received only scant attention. Membrane lipids have, however, been exhaustively studied; generation of the OH$^{\cdot}$ radical is likely to occur close to mitochondrial and microsomal membranes, since these are the intracellular location of high oxygen reduction activity, and membrane phospholipids are the likely primary targets for attack according to the following scheme:

$$R - CH = CH - CH_2 - CH = CH - (CH_2)n - COOH$$

$$\downarrow OH^{\cdot}$$

$$R - CH = CH - CH - CH = CH - (CH_2)_n - COOH$$

$$\downarrow$$

$$R - CH = CH - CH = CH - CH - (CH_2)_n - COOH$$

$$\downarrow O_2$$

$$R- CH = CH - CH = CH - \underset{\overset{|}{O - O^{\cdot}}}{CH} - (CH_2)_n - COOH$$

$$R-H \searrow \downarrow$$

$$R - CH = CH - CH = CH - \underset{\overset{|}{O - OH}}{CH} - (CH_2)_n - COOH$$

In this scheme the molecule RH that intervenes in the last stage is a lipid-soluble antioxidant, usually vitamin E. Thus the second level in the process of protection against free radical damage mentioned earlier, is vitamin E which protects against the proliferation of secondary radical species. If there is a dietary insufficiency of vitamin E then the lipid peroxy radical (the penultimate molecule in the above scheme) may initiate a further attack on another unsaturated fatty acid molecule in much the same way as the attack that is shown initiated by the OH$^\cdot$ radical. The third level of containment comes about because the lipid hydroperoxide product of the above sequence (R-OOH) is not stable but may undergo further iron catalysed degradation, either to a peroxy radical (ROO$^\cdot$) or to an alkoxy radical (RO$^\cdot$). Glutathione peroxidase has another function in this connection in that it can catalyse the following reaction:

$$R - OOH + 2GSH \xrightarrow{GSHpx} R - OH + GSSG + H_2O$$

R - OH can thereafter be further degraded safely and the risk of iron-catalysed degradation of R-OOH is thereby eliminated. Selenium thus has a role to play through glutathione peroxidase in this tertiary protective mechanism. The entire scheme of containment of free radical damage to biological systems thus depends on an adequate dietary supply of Mn, Cu, Zn and vitamin E; ascorbic acid (vitamin C) may be added to this list since it may be involved in the regeneration of vitamin E from the tocopheroxy radical that is formed when vitamin E acts at the last stage of the lipid peroxidation process set out in the above scheme.

(Note: original references have been omitted from this section since the material has been reviewed recently by the present authors. Detailed citations are to be found in references (2-4)).

MICRONUTRIENTS AND TRACE ELEMENTS IN PROTECTION AGAINST CANCER

Among the human diseases in which free radicals may be of significance are ischaemic heart disease and cancer, in some or perhaps all of its multiple forms and aetiologies. The fact that these are the major "Western Killer Disease" has given great impetus to the suggestion that nutritional adequacy may be a major factor in their prevention. Indeed it is true to say that the emotive overtones with which much of the discussion is overlaid are often a disservice to objective scientific evaluation of the significance of nutritional supplementation in the prevention of these diseases. Early work (eg 10) in which low levels of circulating nutrients were found associated with overt disease or following early diagnosis of cancer does little to convince one of the value of good nutrition in disease prevention, since it is not possible to distinguish whether the low level of a nutrient is a cause or a consequence of the disease; the many subsequent similar observations (9) must be viewed in the same light, and the several contradictory observations where a correlation was not found make any conclusion, based on this type of evidence alone, of doubtful validity. Many studies have shown a strong inverse correlation between standardised mortality due to cancer and consumption of foods, which can be calculated from food tables to have a certain level of the nutrients in question (1,5,6). But these studies, which did not include measurement of the levels of the actual nutrients concerned can at best be regarded as indicative of a correlation worthy of further study. Deductions about actual nutrient levels that are derived from food tables are notoriously inaccurate, and, in consideration of the aetiogenesis of cancer where the key events in the pathogenic process may have occurred many years earlier, the food nutrient levels that apply many years later are of little value in evaluating their nutritional significance at the actual time when the pathogenic process was initiated.

New evidence is becoming available that provides a more meaningful database from which deductions and conclusions may be made. This begins to provide quite persuasive epidemiological evidence that a low plasma level of certain nutrients may occur in Western countries and that this is associated with an increased risk of cancer. A prospective study (6) used a cohort of men in Basel, Switzerland whose blood nutrient levels had been measured reliably some years previously, and who are now being followed to record the incidence of all forms of cancer; the published data are thus interim and the study is continuing. The study may be compared with three other studies which are also in progress, in Hawaii (8), at Washington (7) and at Harvard (11).

The overall mortality in the Basel study due to lung and stomach cancer was significantly correlated with low plasma beta-carotene levels, in agreement with the Hawaii and Washington studies. Also, in agreement with the Harvard study, plasma vitamin A was found in the Basel subjects to be significantly lower in men who subsequently died of stomach cancer. Vitamin A and beta-carotene are additional risk factors among the nutrients that need to be considered in this context. Low levels of vitamin C were found in the Basel study to be associated with high incidence of cancer and with other deaths due to nonmalignant causes. A common factor in the Basel and Washington studies was a low mean alpha-tocopheral level in subjects who subsequently died from gastrointestinal cancer and carcinoma of the lung. A new parameter, called the normative cummulative index (NCI) of the antioxidant vitamin E and C, and of beta-carotene, was introduced in the Basel study and the age-standardised mean NCI was found to be significantly depressed as an apparent predisposing factor for all major cancer types.

REFERENCES

1.    Committee on Diet, Nutrition and Cancer.  Diet, Nutrition and Cancer,

104

Washington DC, USA (1982) National Academy Press

2.     Diplock AT (1984) Med Bull 62:78-80

3.     Diplock AT (1987) In: GF Combs, JE Spallholz, OA Levander, JE Oldfield (Eds) Selenium biology and medicineAv New York pp90-103

4.     Diplock AT, Chandhry FA (1988) In: AS Prasad (Ed) Essential and toxic trace elements in human health and disease. Alan R, Liss, New York pp211-226

5.     Doll R and Peto R (1982) J Nat Cancer Inst 66:1191-1208

6.     Gey KF, Brubacher GB, Stahelin HB (1987) Amer J Clin Nutr 45:1368-1377

7.     Menkes MS, Comstock GW, Villeumier JP, Helsing KC, Rider AA, Brookmeyer R (1986) N Eng J Med 315:1250-1254

8.     Nomura AMY, Stemmermann GN, Heilbrun LK, Salkeld RM and Villeumier JP (1985) Cancer Res 45:2369-72

9.     Palmer S (1985) Prog Food Nutr Sci 9:283-341

10.    Shamberger and Frost DV (1969) Canad Med Assoc J 100:682-694

11.    Willett WC, Polk BF and Underwood BA (1985) N Eng J Med 310:430-434

© Elsevier Science Publishers B.V. (Biomedical Division)
Gastric carcinogenesis. P.I. Reed, M.J. Hill, editors.

# SALT AND STOMACH CANCER

JOZEF V JOOSSENS AND HUGO KESTELOOT

Department of Epidemiology, Universitaire Zuikenhuizen Sint-Rafael, Capucinijnenvoer 33, B-3000 Leuven, Belgium

## INTRODUCTION

The role of nutrition in the aetiology of stomach cancer is generally accepted. Problems arise, however, when one has to pinpoint the risk factors for stomach cancer. The classical case-control studies can generate hypotheses about such factors, but their usefulness is limited by the great number of possible risk factors it produces. The hypothesis that salt intake plays an important role in the aetiology of stomach cancer resulted from the analysis of vital statistics (23). This, however, raises other methodological problems, as will be discussed further on.

Although stomach cancer is still the most common cancer worldwide, it is becoming rare in developed countries. Therefore a prospective placebo controlled study of salt intake in the aetiology of stomach cancer is practically impossible because of the costs and the difficulties involved. An alternative is nationwide lowering of salt intake, as occurred in Belgium from 1966 to 1975. It can be monitored at regular intervals and may provide support for the hypothesis (25,31). The different arguments for the salt hypothesis will be reviewed in this chapter.

This chapter is partially based upon a recent paper published in the Proceedings of the Koninklijke Academie voor Geneeskunde van Belgie (Royal Academy of Medicine of Belgium) and reproduced here with courtesy of the Academy.

## METHODS

Truncated mortalities age adjusted to a European population (11) were calculated, using data from a tape of WHO with 10 year age specific death rates. For stomach cancer age-adjusted mortalities were calculated for age groups 45-64 years or 45-74 years, which are the most reliable (24,45). For stroke age group 45-75+ was used, since it was shown that middle-aged stomach cancer death rates gave significant positive correlations in both sexes with all age specific death rates from stroke (in men 45-54 y to 75+, in women 55-64 to 75+) (24).

Yearly mortality trends in percent are calculated from the slope of the linear regression line between the given mortality and time, divided by the average mortality over the same time interval.

## METHODOLOGICAL PROBLEMS

Several scientists still consider mortality statistics as totally unreliable (12).

There are in fact many possible causes of errors:

(1) The size of the diagnostic group is important. The smaller the size, the larger the probability of classification errors. A small number of deaths for a given disease, also increases the possibility of random error, the standard deviation being equal to the square root of the number of deaths. The opposite is also true and eg total mortality is nearly 100% reliable in developed countries, especially near the year of a census count and when total population exceeds 3,000,000.

(2) The size of the population negatively influences the amount of random fluctuation. For a given disease the latter will be large in Luxembourg, Iceland, Malta, etc and small in the USA.

(3) Multiple causes of death may introduce classification errors which are difficult to avoid.

(4) Random diagnostic errors do not affect the mean value, but increase the variance, whereas systematic diagnostic errors produce opposite changes in the means of at least two diagnostic groups. This is exemplified in Belgium by the gradually corrected underclassification of stroke between 1954 and 1968 and by the resulting inverse behaviour of overclassified disease of arteries (24).

(5) Errors are also produced by the changes in the WHO rules, which are occurring every 10 years (6th revision of the International Classification of Diseases in 1948 up to the 9th now).

(6) WHO rules for classification can be applied differently according to the country involved and even according to the region in a given country. Different application of WHO rules with time may also occur.

(7) The use of vital statistics implies the use of heterodemic data (12), ie the deaths are not derived from the same population as the one studied for nutritional data. Heterodemic data are less reliable than hemodemic data, such as eg the "Seven Countries Study" of Ancel Keys et al (39).

How is it then possible to derive any meaningful result from these data? In order to improve the interpretation of such data, one has to study several types of mortality from many countries, from different years, for both sexes and correlate them between and within countries, between means and between trends. Correlations between countries and within countries are independent of one another and, similarly, the mean and the regression slope are mathematically - but not necessarily biologically - independent in each country. Comparison with all causes is also important both for means and trends, since all causes death rates are only subject to (small) random errors. The comparison of two diseases has other advantages. Each disease is caused by a complex set of genetic and environmental factors. Genetic factors will not be discussed here. The sets of environmental risk factors of two diseases may have a common part, the intersection of the sets (Fig.

1). This reduces the number of possible factors involved. Among the aetiological factors some are positive and increase the risk of the disease, others are negative and decrease the risk. Negative (protective) factors are only needed in the presence of positive factors. Potassium does not decrease blood pressure when the sodium intake is low, but could be important when sodium intake is high. Similarly, fibre is not needed to prevent colon cancer when fat intake is low, as in Japan (40), and HDL-cholesterol plays no role when LDL-cholesterol is really low (<2.5 mmol/l) as in Korea, China or Mexico (7,37,38). All this can be compared with a lifejacket which is only needed when one risks falling into water otherwise it is useless.

The quantitative analysis of the relationship between two diseases is also important. If the slope of the regression line obtained between countries is not different from the one over a given time period in a within-country relationship, the common factor in the intersection of the aetiological sets must be either unique or at least preponderant. Such similarity has a very low probability when many factors are involved, because this would imply that the distribution of several factors among many countries is similar to the change of those factors in one country over time, a very unlikely event. As will be seen in the next section the stomach cancer-stroke relationship points to such a unique or preponderant common factor.

STOMACH CANCER AND STROKE

Stomach cancer mortality (age adjusted 45-64 y) has a remarkable relationship with stroke mortality (age adjusted 45 y and over) (23,24,27-30,33,34). This relationship was a chance finding in 1964 (23). In fact it was already observed in Japan in the late fifties, but separately for stroke (15) and stomach cancer (18) and was published only in Japanese. A graphical representation of the mortality from stomach cancer and stroke in 76 large cities, towns and villages of the Miyagi Prefecture in Japan, and derived from those publications (15,18) is given in Fig. 2. Another geographical relationship, between countries, is given for 34 countries in 1973 and for the latest available year (mostly 1984-85) (Figs. 3,4). Another significant between-countries relationship was observed for percent changes in stomach cancer versus percent changes in stroke mortality (Fig. 8 in Ref 29). Nearly 25 years after our first observation many data became available annually making it possible to obtain within-country observations, eg England and Wales (Fig. 5).

In general there are three different periods in a within-country relationship from 1950 (or somewhat later) to now. The first is one of gradual decrease in stomach cancer associated with an increase of stroke mortality. It generally lasts from 1950 to 1955 as seen in England and Wales, the USA, Sweden, West Germany, Norway, Finland, the Netherlands and Canada. This first period was longer in Japan (1950 to

108

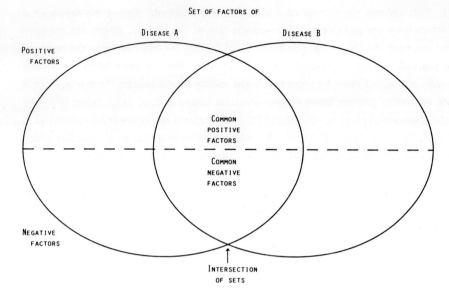

SET OF FACTORS OF

DISEASE A · DISEASE B

POSITIVE
FACTORS

COMMON
POSITIVE
FACTORS

COMMON
NEGATIVE
FACTORS

NEGATIVE
FACTORS

INTERSECTION
OF SETS

Fig. 1. Reproduced by courtesy of the royal Academy of Medicine of Belgium.

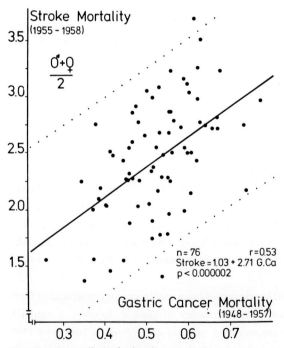

Stroke Mortality
(1955 - 1958)

3.5

$\frac{\male + \female}{2}$

3.0

2.5

2.0

n = 76          r = 0.53
1.5          Stroke = 1.03 + 2.71 G.Ca
p < 0.000002

Gastric Cancer Mortality
(1948 - 1957)

0.3    0.4    0.5    0.6    0.7

Fig. 2. Age adjusted, death rate in large cities, towns and villages
of Miyagi Prefecture, Japan.

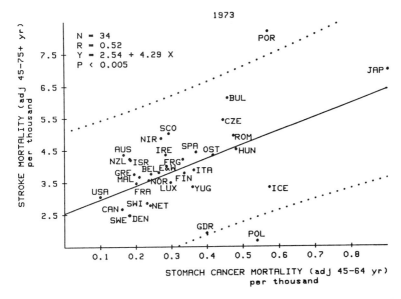

Fig. 3. A between-country relationship in 1973. Reproduced by courtesy of the Royal Academy of Medicine of Belgium

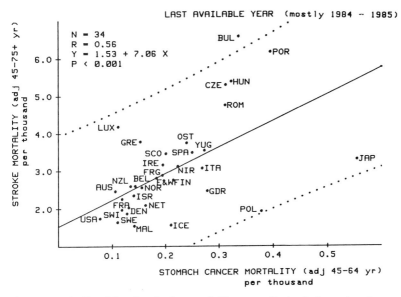

Fig. 4. As in Fig. 3 but for the last available year. Stroke in Japan has decreased much more than expected in relation to stomach cancer, whereas for Bulgaria, Czechoslovakia, Romania and Hungary the opposite has happened. Reproduced by courtesy of the Royal Academy of Medicine of Belgium.

1960), in Belgium (1954 to 1968), in Austria (1955 to 1969), in Scotland (1950 to 1965) and in Australia (1950 to 1970). This phenomenon was not observed in France, Italy or Denmark. It is most likely related to gradual elimination of classification errors, stroke being generally underclassified as already shown in the USA by Acheson (1), and more so in older age groups. In Belgium stroke was classified up to 1968 as diseases of arteries (24). Stomach cancer mortality is always given in the 45-64 y age group and therefore much more reliable (24,45).

The second period shows a linear relationship lasting in most countries until 1973, with both stomach cancer and stroke mortality decreasing regularly at a rate of nearly five cases of stroke for each case of stomach cancer. Representative countries are shown in Figs. 5 to 16.

The third period reflects a much faster decrease of stroke when compared to stomach cancer and is likely related to two confounding factors, the most important being mass treatment of hypertension starting around 1973. The beneficial influence of treatment of hypertension on stroke can be enhanced by an increasing dietary P/S ratio (Polyunsaturated fat/Saturated fat) as observed in the USA, Belgium and Finland where the P/S ratio increased from 0.2 to 0.4-0.6 (17,32,35,36). A much smaller increase occured in England and Wales (36). When, as observed in Hungary, the P/S ratio is decreasing, together with an increasing intake of saturated fat (mostly from butter) it may even reverse the trend and produce an increase of stroke versus a decreasing stomach cancer rate (Fig. 16). The unfavourable influence of a decreasing P/S ratio is a possible reason why stroke mortality decreased much less in Sweden and Denmark than in the USA and Belgium from 1968 to now (Table 1). For Denmark there is good evidence that fat intake has increased over the last fifteen years, whereas in Sweden the changes in nutrition are less clearly defined (14). The most important observation derived from Figures 5 to 16 is that from 1955 to 1973 the slope and intercept of the stomach cancer-stroke regression line are remarkably similar in all countries, except in Belgium where no reliable data existed before 1968, and in Hungary. In six countries (England and Wales, Switzerland, West Germany, the Netherlands, Japan and Italy) the slope values vary between 4.50 and 4.76 and the intercept between 1.65 and 2.87. Therefore, the values of the regression line between 1955 and 1973 in England and Wales can be used to estimate stroke from stomach cancer (or vice versa) during the same period in countries as different as Japan, Hungary, Israel and New Zealand (28). An example of this is given in Fig. 17 where the values for Japan are projected in the regression line derived from England and Wales only (1955 to 1973).

When comparing the 1955-1973 slopes and intercepts from various countries (figs. 5-16) with those obtained between countries in 1973 or in 1985 (Figs. 3-4) the same similarity exists. All this is pointing to a common aetiological factor linking

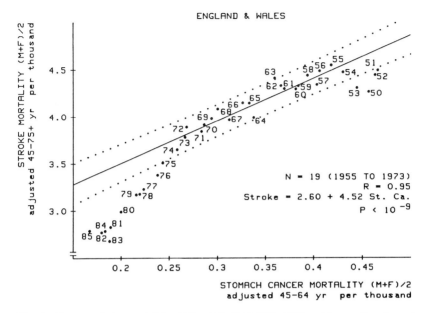

Fig. 5. Three periods are visible: 1950-1955, 1955-1973, 1973 and later. For discussion see text. Updated and reproduced by courtesy of the American Journal of Clinical Nutrition.

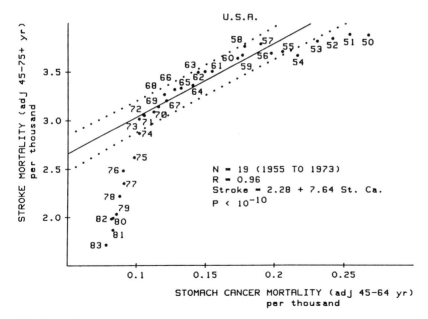

Fig. 6. As in figure 5. Reproduced by courtesy of the Royal Academy of Medicine of Belgium.

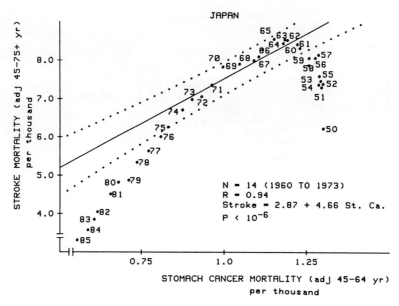

Fig. 7. The first period extends from 1950 to 1960. Reproduced by courtesy of the Royal Academy of Medicine of Belgium.

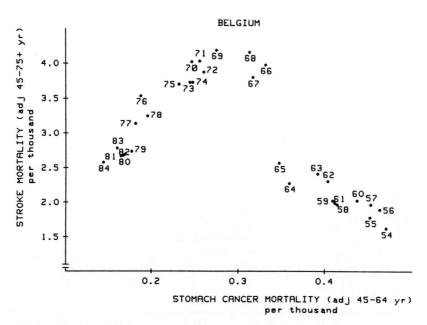

Fig. 8. The first period extends to 1968 and is due to gradual correction of classification errors (24).

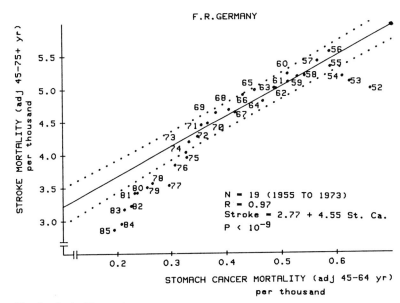

Fig. 9. As in Figure 5.

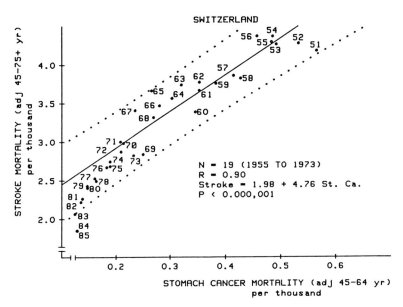

Fig. 10. Only one period (both death rates decreasing) up to 1980, then a near vertical decrease of stroke mortality.

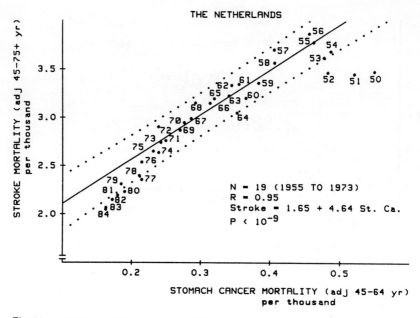

Fig. 11. As in Figure 5, but the last period much less marked.

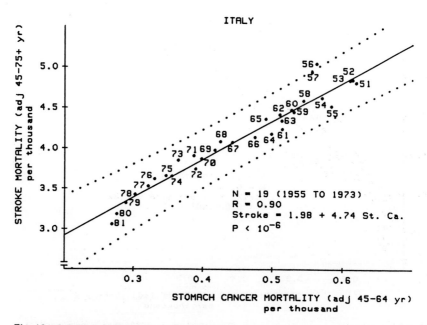

Fig. 12. Only one period visible, both death rates decreasing in a quantitatively similar way as in the other countries.

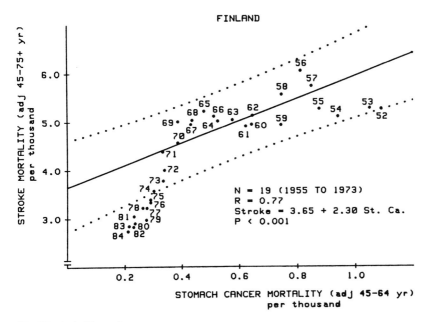

Fig. 13. As in Figure 5.

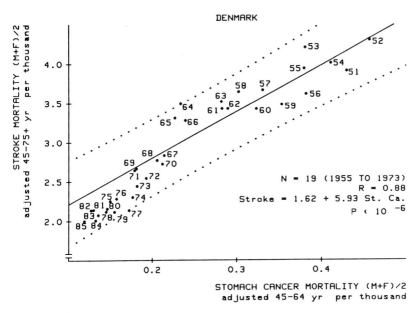

Fig. 14. Only one period visible, with all points lying under the regression line since 1970. Updated and reproduced by courtesy of the American Journal of Clinical Nutrition.

116

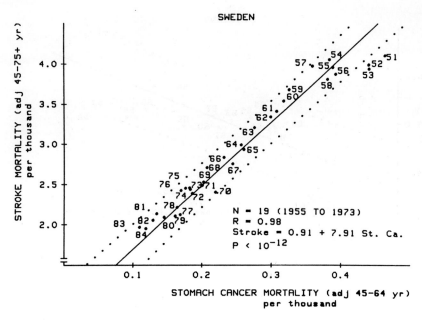

Fig. 15. Only first and second periods visible. Reproduced by courtesy of the Royal Academy of Medicine of Belgium.

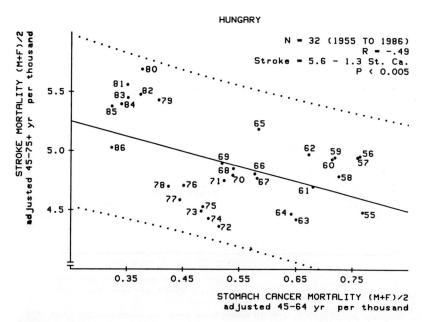

Fig. 16. With marked discontinuity after 1971 and 1978, and probably due to classification changes, there is an overall tendency to increasing stroke with decreasing stomach cancer death rates. This is consistent with increasing all causes mortality (Table 1). Reproduced by courtesy of the Royal Academy of Medicine of Belgium.

TABLE 1

SIGNIFICANT YEARLY PERCENT CHANGE IN MORTALITY (O + O)/2 FROM 1968-69 TO LATEST AVAILABLE YEAR

| | Stomach Cancer | Stroke | All Causes | Ischaemic Heart Disease | Rectal Cancer | Latest Year |
|---|---|---|---|---|---|---|
| England and Wales | -3.4 | -2.7 | -1.2 | -0.4 | -0.5 | 85 |
| USA | -2.7 | -4.6 | -1.6 | -3.7 | -3.9 | 84 |
| Japan | -3.9 | -5.2 | -2.6 | -1.8 | +0.8 | 86 |
| Belgium | -4.3 | -3.4 | -1.4 | -2.0 | -3.2 | 84 |
| West Germany | -4.1 | -2.9 | -1.6 | ns | -2.1 | 86 |
| Switzerland | -4.3 | -3.0 | -1.7 | +0.5 | -2.1 | 86 |
| The Netherlands | -3.4 | -2.6 | -1.0 | -1.3 | -1.6 | 85 |
| Italy | -3.4 | -1.8 | -1.3 | -1.0 | -0.7 | 83 |
| Finland | -4.0 | -3.5 | -2.1 | -1.0 | ns | 86 |
| Denmark | -3.0 | -1.9 | -0.2 | -0.9 | -1.5 | 85 |
| Sweden | -3.7 | -1.8 | -0.8 | -0.8 | ns | 85 |
| Hungary | -3.2 | +1.2 | +0.7 | ns | +2.8 | 86 |

Stomach and rectal cancer are age-adjusted 45-64 y; stroke, all causes and ischemic heart disease 45 to 75+ y. Ischaemic heart disease and rectal cancer trends are added as rough indicators of changes in fat consumption (24).

118

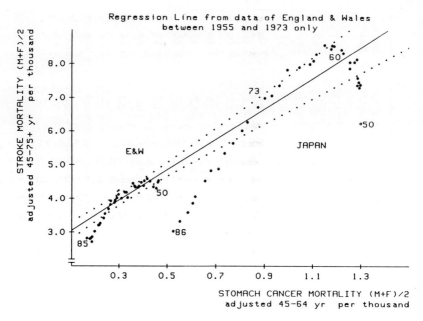

Fig. 17. The data from Figure 5 are extrapolated and those from Japan are projected here upon, showing a striking similarity in behaviour for countries with such different lifestyles. However, this can be explained by decreasing common factors, salt intake, though at a much higher level in Japan (44,56).

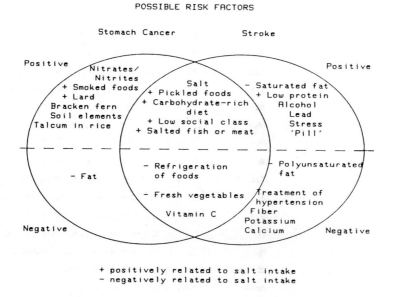

Fig. 18. Reproduced by courtesy of the Royal Academy of Medicine of Belgium.

stomach cancer and stroke. This factor is not necessarily active in the same person. The fact that the correlation between stroke and stomach cancer concerns different age groups (45-75+ versus 45-64 years) is evidence to prove the opposite and this was confirmed in an autopsy study (56).

## THE AETIOLOGY OF STOMACH CANCER

The sets of possible factors as found in the literature for both diseases are given in Fig. 18. All the positive common factors, the intersection of both sets, are directly related to salt intake. Starchy food, whenever found in association with stomach cancer, is always salted. None of the case-control studies was done in a country where the starchy food was not salted. In Nigeria, where salt intake is low (around 100 mmol/day), and carbohydrate intake very high, stomach cancer is low as shown by registry data (11). The inverse relationship between stomach cancer or stroke mortality with social class may be mediated by salt intake. Since salted foods - cured, pickled foods, salted meats and fish, cheese, bread and other cereals, preserves, etc - are at the same time cheaper, a higher salt intake can be expected in lower social classes and this was confirmed in Belgium (26).

The refrigeration of foods is the most important of the negative (protective) factors. There is a consistent relationship between the start of the decrease of stroke and stomach cancer and the mass use of iceboxes, refrigerators and deepfreezes. Both diseases started to decrease in the USA, Australia and New Zealand around 1952-30, in Western Europe after World War II, except Portugal (around 1975), in Japan in 1960, in Eastern Europe between 1960 and 1970 (27,33,34).

The indicated years are consistent with the time of mass introduction of refrigeration techniques in the different countries. Refrigeration of food makes the use of salt for food preservation redundant. It is probably one of the major advances of this century in terms of public health. The use of cooling techniques had other advantages, it reduced the possibility of moulds overgrowing the food (4) and in cured, pickled foods it made the conversion of nitrates into nitroso-carcinogens more difficult (55). The latter two properties, however, have no influence in stroke mortality, they are outside the intersection of the aetiological data sets. In Japan a higher milk intake was singled out as a protective factor (19). This is quite possible, since milk in Japan was an indicator of a less traditional, less salted food intake. In Finland, with one of the highest milk intakes in the world, but coupled with a very high salt intake, stomach cancer was nearly as high as in Japan, namely in 1952 1.1% in Finland and 1.3% in Japan (45-64 y, ($\male$ + $\female$)/2). Vegetables are protective, especially the yellow and green varieties (20). Vitamin C is not related to salt in itself, but one of the major sources of vitamin C is found in vegetables (potatoes, etc) or fruits. It may act by inhibiting the conversion of nitrate/nitrite into

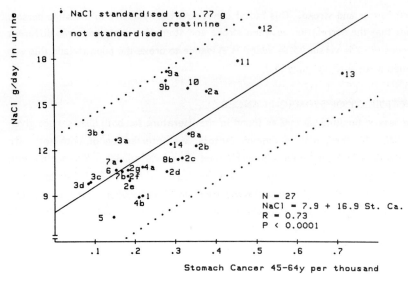

l=Netherlands,78; 2=North of Belgium,66-83; 3=US,61-77; 4=E&W,78-78
5=France,77; 6=New Zealand,75; 7=Australia,73-74; 8=FRG,73-76; 9=Finland,77-79
10=Scotland,72; 11=Portugal,78; 12=Bulgaria,70; 13=Japan,79; 14=Italy,79

Fig. 19. 24h NaCl excretion estimated from observed stomach cancer death rates. The references for the salt excretion values are given in (27), except for France (10), Japan (22), Italy (50), the Netherlands (54) and Belgium 1983 (31).

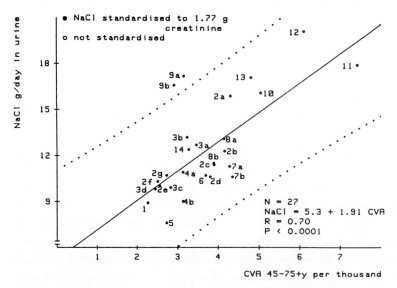

l=Netherlands,78; 2=North of Belgium,66-83; 3=US,61-77; 4=E&W,78-78
5=France,77; 6=New Zealand,75; 7=Australia,73-74; 8=FRG,73-76; 9=Finland,77-79
10=Scotland,72; 11=Portugal,78; 12=Bulgaria,70; 13=Japan,79; 14=Italy,79

Fig. 20. As in Figure 19, but now estimated from stroke mortality.

carcinogens (43,55) and also by the fact that fresh vegetables or fruits are less or not salted. Epidemiologically the average salt intake in a population can be estimated from its stroke and stomach cancer mortality levels (Fig. 19-20). In both cases the intercept is significantly different from zero. For stroke the relationship was also significant, at least, some years ago. Major confounding factors such as treatment for hypertension and changing fat intake may obscure the picture now. The Intersalt data, which will be available soon, may clarify this problem.

The evidence from case-control studies is not as clear, with many nutritional factors found as of possible importance (see Reference 46). Nevertheless, the foods which are singled out most frequently were salted, cured and pickled foods, making it, however, difficult to decide which factor is more important the salt or the nitrate/nitrite content. Recent evidence from Chile and England and Wales have pointed out that nitrates, mostly from fresh vegetables, are probably not important in the aetiology of stomach cancer (2,3,13).

Salt in hypertonic solution has caustic properties, injuring the taste buds (6), the skin from salt miners (42) or from lobster fishermen (5) and, experimentally, the stomach mucosa in mice. Hypertonic salt solutions occur more easily with salt than with other products, since salt is totally ionized and at the same time the smallest molecule present in nutrition in gram amounts.

Experimentally it was shown that hypertonic salt in the stomach:

(1) Induced, in a dose-response relationship, DNA and ornithine decarboxylase synthesis in a similar way as nitroso-carcinogens (16).

(2) Enhanced the carcinogenic action of nitrosamides such as MNNG (N-Methyl-N-nitro-N'-nitroso-guanidine), being thereby co-carcinogenic (51,52).

(3) Had a significant promoting activity for stomach cancer, when given after the administration of a carcinogen (51).

In line with those findings the prevalence of atrophic gastritis is or was very common in countries with a high salt intake as in Japan (47,58), Colombia (9,44) or Finland (48). Chronic atrophic gastritis was more prevalent in high risk areas of Colombia than in low risk areas (9). In Japan it was shown that, among 414 inhabitants of the Akita Prefecture, a significant correlation existed between salt intake and intestinal metaplasia of the stomach (57). In Belgium a case-control study showed that stomach cancer patients added significantly more salt to their food than controls (53).

The still hypothetical aetiology of stomach cancer can then be summarized as follows. Hypertonic salt solution in the stomach delays the emptying of the stomach by closing the pylorus following the activation of the duodenal osmoreceptors (21). Hypertonic salt solution in the stomach damages the stomach mucosa, causing first hypertrophic gastritis, then atrophic gastritis and finally intestinal metaplasia (8).

This damage is more pronounced in the antral part of the stomach in relation with our upright position. The pH of the stomach rises with the atrophy of the stomach mucosa and although this inhibits partially the formation of nitroso-carcinogens it increases the conversion of nitrates to nitrites by bacterial overgrowth. Nitrates in the food, especially from cured foods, may at this stage increase the risk of stomach cancer. If the experimental results may be extrapolated to the human being, which has not been demonstrated as yet, the high salt content of the stomach may exert co-carcinogenic and promotional activity.

Recently interesting data became available from the Peoples Republic of China (41). In the province of Henan there is a significant rank correlation between the incidence of stomach cancer and the quantity of salt sold in 108 counties and cities (0.63 for men and 0.54 for women). The average amount of salt sold per person in the higher incidence areas was 21 g/day compared with 16 g/day in the lower incidence areas with extremes of more than 22 g/day and less than 11 g/day.

Finally, in Belgium and Switzerland the results of the salt intake reduction are interesting. In Belgium the naturally occurring decrease in salt intake (increasing affluence, refrigerators, etc) was enhanced by a nationwide public health education campaign (31). The campaign aimed at a reduction of salt and saturated fat, together with an increase in polyunsaturated fat. Between 1966 and 1975 the 24h urinary salt excretion gradually decreased from about 240 to 160 mmol/24h. Afterwards only minor changes occurred (25,31). Stomach cancer and stroke mortality started to decrease faster in both the north and the south of Belgium around 1972 and levelled off after 1979 suggesting a lag time of 4-5 years for both diseases. During the period 1968-1980 the decrease in stomach cancer and stroke mortality was highest in Belgium among the common market partners (31). Of course, the favourable change in the P/S ratio may also have influenced this result. On the other hand, salt intake being higher in the north of Belgium, a markedly higher stomach cancer mortality was observed there (35). This was not confirmed for stroke mortality, the latter being higher in the south of Belgium, but the P/S ratio is now around 0.5-0.6 in the north, rising from 0.2 in 1960, versus 0.3-0.4 in the south of Belgium (35), and this may as observed elsewhere act as a confounding factor.

A marked, unconscious (not produced by an anti-salt campaign) decrease in iodized salt intake was observed in Switzerland from 1951 to 1976. That the decrease was not spurious was indicated by the fact that the Swiss government had to double the iodine content of the salt in 1962 (49). No further drop in stomach cancer has been observed since 1981 (Fig. 10), consistent with a 5 year lag time. From the observed changes in stomach cancer or stroke mortality (1951 to 1976, see Figure 10) one can calculate the difference in salt intake using the equations from

Figures 19 and 20. The estimated difference is respectively 6.4 and 4.2 g salt/day compared with the observed difference in sales of iodized salt of 6.3 g/day (49).

## SUMMARY

All chronic degenerative diseases and especially chronic cardiovascular diseases and cancer have a complex multifactorial origin. The aetiological factors of a given disease constitute a set of factors. When comparing stroke and stomach cancer there are two sets of factors with the common factors at the intersection of the sets. The comparison of different causes of death under different conditions (sex, age groups, average mortality, mortality trends, all between and within countries) improves the interpretation of mortality data, making spurious associations unlikely, and makes it possible to derive meaningful conclusions.

Evidence is given that stroke and stomach cancer are linked through a high salt intake, with refrigeration of foods, fresh vegetables or fruits, and vitamin C as possible protective factors. Confounding factors are mostly acting on stroke mortality, such as better mass treatment of hypertension and a changing P/S ratio of the fats in food. The possible role of nitrate/nitrite from food in the aetiology of stomach cancer was discussed.

Since the nutritional recommendations for preventing stroke and stomach cancer are quite similar a prudent diet should include a gradual decrease of salt intake. Monitoring of the changes in diet and mortality in different populations is necessary in order to validate the recommendations.

## ACKNOWLEDGEMENTS

FWGO (Brussels) and the ASLK (Brussels) provided the funds. The aid of J Geboers for the mortality data was highly appreciated. L Cooreman and G De Vadder were of considerable help for the references. J Rongy typed and R Struyven corrected the text. C Lauwereys made the figures. To all of them my most sincere thanks.

## REFERENCES

1.  Acheson RM (1966) In: Kost K (ed). Cerebrovascular Disease Epidemiology. Publ Hlth Monogr 76, DHEW, Washington, pp23-40

2.  Al-Dabbagh S, Forman D, Bryson D, Stratton I, Doll R (1986) Br J Indust Med 43:507-515

3.  Armijo R, Gonzalez A, Orellana M, Coulson AH, Sayre JW, Detels R (1981) Int J Epidemiol 10:57-62

4.  Avery-Jones F (1967) Recent Adv Gastroenterol 1:93-98

5.  Beer WE, Jones M, Eifion Jones W (1968) Br Med J 1:807-809

6.  Blais CA, Pangborn RM, Borhani NO, Ferrell MF, Prineas RJ, Laing B (1986)

124

Am J Clin Nutr 44:232-243

7. Conner WE, Cerqueira MT, Connor RW, Wallace RB, Manilow MR, Casdorph HR (1978) Am J Clin Nutr 31:1131-1142

8. Correa P (1983) In: Sherlock P, Morson BC, Barbara L, Veronesi U (eds). Precancerous Lesions of the Gastrointestinal Tract. Raven press, New York pp145-153

9. Correa P, Cuello C, Duque E, Burbano LC, Garcia FT, Bolanos O, Brown C, Haenszel W (1976) J Natl Cancer Inst 57:1027-1035

10. Cottet J (1981) Bull Acad R Med Belg 136:556-565

11. Doll R, Muir C, Waterhouse I (1970) Cancer incidence in five continents. Vol. II. Springer Verlag, Berlin, FRG.

12. Feinstein AR (1986) Clinical Epidemiology. Holt-Saunders International, Eastbourne

13. Forman D, Al-Dabbagh S, Doll R (1985) Nature 313:620-625

14. Frank J (1987) UK and international food consumption patterns. Vol. 3. In: International Dietary Trends (Review paper). Horton Publishing Ltd, Bradford

15. Fujisaku S, Ito T, Kamoi M, Hiraide H (1960) Tohoku Igaku Zasshi 61:628-634

16. Furihata C, Sato Y, Hosaka M, Matsushima T, Furukawa F, Takahashi M (1984) Biochem Biophys Res Commun 121:1027-1032

17. Goor R, Hosking JD, Dennis BH, Graves KL, Waldman GT, Haynes SG (1985) Am J Clin Nutr 41:299-311

18. Hiraide H (1959) Tohoku Igaku Zasshi 59:286-293

19. Hirayama T (1967) In: Harris (ed). Proceedings of the 9th International Cancer Congress, Tokyo, 1966, UICC Monograph Series 10. Springer Verlag, Berlin, pp27-48

20. Hirayama T (1985) In: Joossens JV, Hill MJ, Geboers J (eds). Diet and Human Carcinogenesis, International Congress Series 685. Excerpta Medica, Amsterdam, pp191-198

21. Hunt JN, Pthak JD (1960) J Physiol 154:254-269

22. Ikeda M, Kasahara M, Koizumi A, Watanabe T (1986) Prev Med 15:46-59

23. Joossens JV (1965) Verh Kon Vlaam Akad Geneeskd Belg 27:489-545

24. Joossens JV (1980) In: Kesteloot H, Joossens JV (eds). Epidemiology of Arterial Blood Pressure. Martinus Nijhoff Publishers, The Hague, pp489-508

25. Joossens JV (1988) Nutr Rev 46:100-104

26. Joossens JV, Claessens J, Geboers J, Claes JH (1980) In: Kesteloot H, Joossens JV (eds). Epidemiology of Arterial Blood pressure. Martinus Nijhoff, The Hague, pp45-63

27. Joossens JV, Geboers J (1981) Nutr Cancer 2:250-261

28. Joossens JV, Geboers J (1983) In: Sherlock P (ed). Precancerous Lesions of the Gastrointestinal Tract. Raven Press, New York, pp97-113

29. Joossens JV, Geboers J (1984) In: Levin B, Riddell RH (eds). Frontiers of Gastrointestinal Cancer. Elsevier Science Publishing Co, New York, pp167-183

30. Joossens JV, Geboers J (1985) In: Joossens JV, Hill MJ, Geboers J (eds). Diet and Human Carcinogenesis, International Congress Series 685. Excerpta Medica, Amsterdam, pp277-297

31. Joossens JV, Geboers J (1985) In: Bulpitt CJ (ed). Epidemiology of hypertension. Elsevier, Amsterdam

32. Joossens JV, Geboers J (1985) In: Kaplan RM, Criqui MH (eds). Behavioral Epidemiology and Disease Prevention, NATO ASI Series A: Life Sciences, Vol. 84. Plenum, New York, pp103-120

33. Joossens JV, Geboers J (1986) Biomed and Pharmacother 40:127-138

34. Joossens JV, Geboers J (1987) Am J Clin Nutr 45:1277-1288

35. Joosens JV, Geboers J, Kesteloot H (1985) Verh K Acad Geneeskd Belg 47:207-244

36. Katan MR, Beynen AC (1981) Lancet 2:371

37. Kesteloot H, Huang DX, Yang XS, Claes J, Rosseneu M, Geboers J, Joossens JV (1985) Arteriosclerosis 5:427-433

38. Kesteloot H, Lee CS, Park HM, Kegels C, Geboers J, Claes JH, Joossens JV (1982) Circulation 65(4):795-799

39. Keys A (1980) Seven Countries: A Multivariate Analysis of Death and Coronary Heart Disease. Harvard University Press, Cambridge (MA)

40. Kuratsune M, Honda T, Englyst HN, Cummings JH (1986) Jpn J Cancer Res (Gann) 77:736-738

41. Lu JB, Qin YM (1987) China. Int J Epid 16:171-176

42. Meyer P (1982) L'homme et le sel: reflexions sur l'histoire humaine et l'evolution de la medecine. Editions Fayard, Paris

43. Mirvish SS (1975) Am NY Acad Sci 258:175-180

44. Montes G, Cuello C, Correa P, Zarama G, Liuzza G, Zavala D, de Marin E, Haenszel W (1985) J Cancer Res Clin Oncol 109:42-45

45. Peto R (1986) In: Hallgren B, et al (eds). Diet and Prevention of Coronary Heart Disease and Cancer. Raven Press, New York pp1-16

46. Risch HA, Jain M, Choi NW, Fodor JG, Pfeiffer CJ, Howe GR, Harrison LW, Crab KJ, Miller AB (1985) Am J Epidemiol 122:947-959

47. Sasaki N (1964) Geriatrics 19:735-744

48. Siurala M, Isokoski K, Varis K, Kekki M (1968) Scand J Gastroenterol 3:211-223

49. Societe des Salines Suisses de Rhin Reunies (1978) La situation actuelle du sel iode en Suisse. Schweizerhalle, Switzerland, pp1-18

50. Strazzullo P, Trevisan M, Farinaro E, Cappuccio FP, Ferrara LA, De Campora E, Mancini M (1983) Eur Heart J 4:608-613

51. Takahashi M, Hasegawa R (1986) In: Hayashi Y, Nagao M, Sugimura T, Takayama S, Tomatis L, Wattenberg LW, Wogan GN (eds). Nutrition and Cancer. Japan Sci Soc Press, Tokyo: VNU Sci Press, Utrecht, pp169-182

52. Tatematsu M, Takahashi M, Fukushima S, Hananouchi M, Shirai T (1975) J Natl Cancer Inst 55:101-106

53. Tuyns A (1988) Salt and gastric intestinal cancer. Submitted for publication

54. Van Binsbergen JJ (1985) Personal communication

55. Weisburger JH, Marquardt H, Mower JH, Hirota N, Mori H, Williams G (1980) Prev Med 9:352-361

56. Whelton PK, Goldblatt P (1982) Am J epidemiol 15:418-427

126

57.    Yamakawa H (1986) Gan No Rinsho 32(6):681-691
58.    Yoshitoshi Y (1967) In: Proceedings of the 3rd World Congress of Gastroenterology, vol. I. Nankodo, Tokyo, pp179-185

© *Elsevier Science Publishers B.V. (Biomedical Division)*
*Gastric carcinogenesis. P.I. Reed, M.J. Hill, editors.*

PRECANCEROUS LESIONS OF THE STOMACH PHENOTYPIC CHANGES AND THEIR DETERMINANTS

PELAYO CORREA

Department of Pathology, Louisiana State University Medical Center, 1901 Perdido Street, New Orleans, LA 70112, USA

The realization that most gastric carcinomas (intestinal type) are preceded by profound changes in the gastric mucosa has led to concerted efforts to study their precancerous process. Different investigators have focussed on different markers and described a wealth of phenotypic changes in the pre-neoplastic state. We will attempt a holistic approach in an effort to interpret the biological process in general, point to gaps in our knowledge which hinder our understanding of the phenomenon, attempts to identify the site of action of the known aetiological factors in the chain of events, examine the clinical significance of the present state of the art and comment on possible future research approaches.

ARCHITECTURAL AND CYTOLOGICAL CHANGES

There seems to be a consensus that the first events which can be linked to the precancerous process are the chronic inflammatory changes in the gastric mucosa. There are several types of chronic gastritis (5), but only those leading to permanent gland loss (i.e. atrophy) have been aetiologically linked to gastric cancer (6). There are 2 types of atrophic gastritis. Autoimmune (Type A) gastritis is practically limited to Scandinavians and is apparently decreasing in incidence. Multifocal (Type B, type AB or pangastritis) is by far the most common type, highly prevalent in all populations displaying high gastric cancer risk. Reflux gastritis associated with previous gastrectomy is statistically associated with gastric cancer. Most of those carcinomas, however, appear in the anastomosis site and are preceded by polyps and cysts which may express poorly understood pathogenic mechanisms which may not be related to the gastrtic changes seen in the gastric mucosa proper.

In chronic atrophic gastritis epithelial cells and glands are lost repeatedly over a span of many years. They are replaced by cells with intestinal phenotype, as discussed by Dr Filipe in this monograph (10). In this process the adult gastric epithelial cell is replaced by another adult cell, a metaplastic intestinal cell. This transformation from gastric to intestinal cells seems to be gradual, as shown by the existence of cells which display gastric and intestinal types of mucin, identified histochemically (22) and ultrastructurally (23). After the transformation is complete, further changes appear in some metaplastic cells which express sulphomucins, a product normally seen in the large but not in the small intestine (Type III or colonic metaplasia). Sulphomucins and "colonic" metaplasias are frequently observed around carcinomas (34) and in the areas of the stomach where metaplasia appears first, like the lesser curvature of the antrum (15). This can be interpreted as indicative of a more advanced stage of metaplasia.

More profound architectural disorganization and nuclear abnormalities are seen in dysplasia, mostly in a background of intestinal metaplasia, suggesting that it represents yet another phenotypic change occurring in cells which had experienced the previous changes (8,14).

## DIGESTIVE ENZYMES

The only digestive enzyme present in the normal stomach is pepsin, active in the initial stages of the digestion of proteins. The precursors of pepsin (zymogen) are the pepsinogens which comprise a heterogeneous group of proteins which fall into two broad groups. Pepsinogen I (PG I) is found mainly in the chief cells of the corpus and fundus mucosa and to a lesser degree in the "neck" cells which are the only normal gastric epithelial cells capable of replication. (The neck cells are multipotential and replicate to replace loss of differentiated cells which produce mucins if located at the faveolar surface or pepsinogen if located deep in the glands). Pepsinogen II (PG II), although stainable in chief cells and neck cells, is abundant in the antral ("pyloric") glands and in the glands of the cardial mucosa (morphologically similar to the antral glands) (31,36). Intestinal metaplasia cells usually do not secrete pepsinogens but dysplasia and carcinoma cells may (mostly PG II), usually in a "patchy" and irregular way. This may be taken as an indication that intestinal metaplasia is a collateral phenomenon which is not in the mainstream of the genomic precancerous changes ("paraneoplastic"). Morphological observations, however, postulate that most dysplasias originate in previously metaplastic cells (8,14). This leads to an alternative explanation of the phenomenon: the pepsinogens disappear when normal gastric cells are replaced by phenotypically mature intestinal cells ("small intestinal metaplasia") but reappear when the phenotype reverts back to a more primitive (dysplastic) cell, equivalent to the "neck" cell of the gastric mucosa which has the capacity to synthesize pepsinogens. Most PG positive carcinomas express PG II, probably indicating some relation to antral glands. An elevated PG II level may be indicative of gastric cancer, but a low level does not preclude such a diagnosis.

The battery of digestive enzymes normally found in the small intestine are present in small intestinal metaplasia: sucrase, trehalase, leucine aminopeptidase, alkaline phosphatase. This fact has been well documented in humans and has given rise to the denomination of "complete" to this variety of metaplasia. Most of those enzymes are missing in colonic ("incomplete") metaplasia, frequently accompanied by dysplasia or small carcinomas in other areas of the gastric mucosa (21,22). When comparing well advanced with less advanced metaplasia cases, the impression is gained that some enzymes disappear early in the process (i.e. sucrase) while others are found in advanced cases, even if in small amounts (leucineaminopeptidase).

## ANTIGENS

Linking the expression of gastrointestinal antigens to gastric carcinogenesis in humans is not a recent idea. Polyclonal antibodies produced with human colon and normal adult rat stomachs bind to normal human foetal stomach; the intestinal component disappears soon after birth but reappears in metaplasia and neoplasia. The gastric antigen persists throughout adult life but shows a tendency to be depleted when metaplasia and neoplasia make their appearance (9).

Blood group related antigens have been "mapped" in the gastrointestinal mucosa (4,24) and special interest has been given to Lewis[a] (Le[a]), which is present in the normal foetal stomach but absent in the normal adult stomach. Monoclonal antibodies against Le[a] have been detected in the serum of patients with gastric carcinoma (17). The prevalence of such antibodies in the antral mucosa in gastric biopsies has been reported as follows: normal = 0% (0/37); grade 1 atrophy = 18% (2/11); grade 2 atrophy = 31% (5/16); grade 3 atrophy (intestinal metaplasia) = 61% (8/13); grade 4 atrophy (advanced metaplasia) = 100% (3/3). The pattern reflects a gradual increase of the foetal antigen expression as the precancerous process advances.

Mucus associated antigens have been detected in gastric cancer and intestinalized gastric mucosa (1,27). Three main antigenic groups associated with goblet cells have been described. M3SI (small intestine) and M3D (duodenum) have been observed in intestinal metaplasia of "benign" gastric mucosa. M3C (colon) as well as M3D and M3SI were found in metaplasia adjacent to gastric carcinomas. The latter pattern is similar to foetal duodenum which led to the postulate that as metaplasia advances, although it resembles colonic mucosa on morphologic grounds, it may really be expressing the phenotype of foetal duodenum (28).

Other well known embryonal antigens have been detected in gastric carcinomas as well as in intestinal metaplasia and dysplasia. Such is the case of carcino-embryonic antigen (CEA) (29) and alfa-foeto protein (AFP) (18). In addition to the above, other antigens are shared by cancer cells and intestinalized cells surrounding the tumour. Such is the case for pregnancy-specific beta-glycoprotein (SP-1), beta chorionic gonadotrophin (B-HCG) and human placental lactogen (HPL). Metaplastic cells not associated with cancer do not express these antigens, but the two types of metaplasia with contrasting antigen expressions are not distinguishable on morphologic grounds alone (35).

A murine fibrosarcoma associated antigen which is expressed in foetal but not adult gastrointestinal tissue (YFA) was studied in conjunction with H$^3$ thymidine labelling in gastric mucosal biopsies showing chronic atrophic gastritis and intestinal metaplasia. There was a remarkable coincidence between the increased thymidine labelling and the expression of the foetal antigens. Very few studies have been made in which two separate markers of pre-malignant changes are observed in the same cell compartment. In these experiments synchrony between the two phenotypic changes is apparent (19). A human second trimester foetal antigen has been found increasingly expressed as the precancerous process advances: 10% in superficial gastritis, 38% in chronic atrophic gastritis, 50% in intestinal metaplasia and 86% in dysplasia (13).

## ONCOGENE EXPRESSION

A few studies have shown that foci of intestinal metaplasia of the gastric mucosa express oncogene products. Noguchi et al have reported elevated p21 ras oncogene product in metaplastic cells (30). Ciclitira et al reported increased expression of the p62 product of the c-myc oncogene in inflammatory, metaplastic and dysplastic gastric mucosa. Some expression was also found in the epithelial cells of the mucus neck region (3). Products of the ras gene expression may be associated with cellular transformation while product of myc gene may reflect excessive replication.

## SYNCHRONY

When the different components of the phenotype are studied (architecture, nuclear morphology, enzymes, mucins, antigen expression, etc), synchrony is found only in the most general sense. In most "advanced" cases in which dysplastic or neoplastic changes are found in some area of the mucosa, the metaplastic changes are extensive, the architecture resembles the colonic mucosa, the digestive enzymes are absent, sulphomucin is present and embryonal or foetal antigens are expressed. But when "synchrony" is looked for in more refined steps, many unexpected results are obtained: the loss of digestive enzymes is somewhat irregular and does not always match the architectural or mucin findings: sialo and sulphomucins not always match morphology in intestinal metaplasia; mature and "immature" antigens may be found in advanced dysplasia, etc. It is entirely possible that the genetic make-up of the subject and the intensity or frequency of the individual components of environmental insults determine the pattern of phenotypic changes. Hopefully, future investigation will throw light into this apparently confused state of affairs.

Most investigators agree that the gastric pre-neoplastic process manifests itself in humans not as an "all or none" phenomenon but as a gradual transition from the mature to the embryonal phenotype. This lack of "instancy" in the phenotypic change may be a problem when classifying metaplasia as a mutation.

It seems safe to postulate that in the gastric precancerous process several broad steps can be identified:

a.   In the initial stages, characterized by excessive cell death, regeneration and atrophy, the epithelial cells preserve their normal adult gastric phenotype.

b.   When the above cells are replaced by intestinal cells, the adult phenotype of the small intestine predominates.

c.   In situations which imply a higher gastric cancer risk (older individuals, presence of dysplasia) or when small cancers are detected, the metaplastic cells do not reproduce adult small intestinal cells. They morphologically resemble large intestine and express products reminiscent of foetal tissues.

d.   The most advanced stages display an immature phenotype and secrete products of foetal nature or mixed phenotypic characteristics which in the normal adult stomach are only found in the neck cells.

These apparently gradual changes may be interpreted as a gradual loss of differentiation leading to a primitive-type cell. Since it is possible to identify these steps, it becomes important to examine at which step the known aetiological agents are operating.

## TIMING OF AETIOLOGICAL FACTORS

The present state of the art makes it possible to explore specific aetiological agents and their effects on specific points in the chain of causation. The factors so far identified fall in three main categories; irritants, mutagens and insufficient intake of protective agents, mainly micronutrients. The following are preliminary results of our work in this area.

### Irritants

Salt is the most prevalent recognized irritant of the gastric mucosa, but others very prevalent are alcohol, aspirin and probably Campylobacter pylori.

We have correlated gastric biopsy findings in the Colombia (Narino) population with sodium excretion in terms of urinary sodium/creatinine ratio, previously shown to be a reliable index for group comparisons (22). Table 1 shows the odds ratios (relative risk) for the main categories of gastric histology and the 95% confidence intervals.

In Table 1, odds ratios were adjusted for age, sex, pH and nitrite content of gastric juice in a logistic regression analysis. Sodium/creatinine ratios were dichotomized at the point of the median value (2). The data show that excessive salt intake significantly exerts its action in two specific points of the chain: it induces atrophy and has a role in the induction of dysplasia (lower confidence intervals above 1). These results are very much in line with experimental work on gastric atrophy (16) and MNNG-induced carcinogenesis (37). Surprisingly, salt does not appear to play a role in superficial gastritis. Recent findings suggest that Campylobacter infection may be the overriding factor in superficial gastritis (20). The role of salt in inducing metaplasia is not apparent in the present study. The slightly elevated but not statistically significant relative risk is compatible with a lack of effect or with a secondary weak effect, perhaps depending on other factors. Intestinal metaplasia represents a radical genotypic change in the cells (mutation?) not expected from salt alone, but it is possible that salt facilitates the action of a true mutagen.

TABLE 1

ODDS RATIOS OF GASTRIC LESIONS BY SODIUM/CREATININE (S/C) RATIO

| Diagnosis | S/C 4.88 | 4.88 | O.R. (Adjusted) | (95% C.I.) |
|---|---|---|---|---|
| Normal | 40 | 39 | 1.0 | |
| Superficial gastritis | 32 | 35 | 0.87 | (0.45 - 1.70) |
| Chronic atrophic gastritis | 28 | 13 | 2.50 | (1.09 - 5.77) |
| Intestinal metaplasia | 36 | 28 | 1.57 | (0.76 - 3.28) |
| Dysplasia | 9 | 3 | 7.24 | (1.14 - 45.84) |

Mutants

Since we do not know which mutants are relevant in high risk human populations, we cannot test directly their effects. Intragastric nitrosation as a source of mutants has not been proven but remains a viable possibility. The leading candidates as N-nitroso-carcinogens at the present time are the mutagen-carcinogen(s) in nitrosated Japanese fish (not yet chemically identified) (39) and the nitroso-indoles (38,40). Excessive nitrite in the gastric juice may be a surrogate for such mutagens, and we have examined its statistical association with gastric precursor lesions in the Narino population, as shown in Table 2.

In Table 2 odds ratios were adjusted for age, sex, sodium/creatinine ratio and addition of salt to food on the table in a logistic regression model. As can be seen, the effect of nitrite is only significant for intestinal metaplasia and dysplasia (lower confidence intervals above 1). These findings make sense in that these are the only steps which require inheritable DNA damage (mutation or expression of repressed genes).

TABLE 2

ODDS RATIOS OF GASTRIC LESIONS BY NITRITE PRESENCE IN GASTRIC JUICE

| Diagnosis | $NO_2$ Detectable | Not Detectable | O.R. (Adjusted) | (95% C.I.) |
|---|---|---|---|---|
| Normal | 73 | 6 | 1.0 | |
| Superficial gastritis | 55 | 12 | 2.64 | (0.77 - 9.06) |
| Chronic atrophic gastritis | 34 | 7 | 3.14 | (0.76 - 13.02) |
| Intestinal metaplasia | 43 | 21 | 3.98 | (1.22 - 12.98) |
| Dysplasia | 7 | 5 | 23.58 | (1.85 - 300.86) |

Protective Agents

At the present time the most consistent evidence in this regard is the inverse association between intake of fresh fruits and vegetables and the risk of gastric cancer and chronic atrophic gastritis (7,11). Fresh fruits and vegetables contain a wealth of micronutrients and non-nutrient compounds whose potential role in disease prevention is mostly unexplored. Preliminary observations hold two groups of compounds as promising: vitamin C and carotenoids. A third group, the tocopherols, may also hold some promise. Work on non-nutrients is pointing to promising compounds, some of which, namely the protease inhibitors, exert a more permanent protection than the antioxidants. Our brief comments will refer only to vitamin C and the carotenoids.

Vitamin C is an excellent blocker of nitrosation and as such should protect against in situ synthesis of N-nitroso carcinogenesis in the stomach. This blocking effect is well documented in vitro, as is its blocking of the synthesis of the non-carcinogen N-nitrosoproline in humans. Epidemiologic studies have found a protective effect against chronic gastritis in some high risk populations (7). The evidence on vitamin C is, therefore, inconclusive at the present time. It is possible that it plays a prominent role in some populations but not in others.

Our studies in the Narino population of Colombia have shown a strong association between low levels of carotenoids and gastric dysplasia but not in any of the other precursor states (12). Therefore, it appears that the effect of this important anti-oxidant is specifically timed for the last step in the precancerous chain of events. This effect in humans is very similar to what has been found experimentally in rats fed MNNG and carotenoids in that the early stages of the process (including metaplasia) are not affected but the last step is inhibited. In addition to beta carotene, the inhibition was also achieved with canthaxanthin, a carotenoid which is not a retinol precursor (32). Recent evidence is accumulating to show that carotenoids exert a protective effect as antioxidants, independent of retinol (vitamin A).

## CLINICAL SIGNIFICANCE AND RESEARCH STRATEGIES

The key to the clinical usefulness of precancerous markers is to identify those that are relevant and applicable to large populations. This information should be obtained by epidemiologic techniques, and they fall in three general categories.

a. Retrospective (case-control) studies in which previous gastric biopsies are available for patients who developed gastric cancer, compared to patients who had previous biopsies but who have not developed cancer. The difficulties of this approach are obvious (the scarcity of patients in each category), but some successful attempts are on record (26).

b. Prospective (cohort) studies in which patients are followed over time after the markers are identified in gastric biopsies. Given the relatively low incidence of gastric cancer in the population, the time involved and the large number of subjects required for significant results, this appraoch appears unrealistic at the present time.

c. Chemoprevention. In this approach markers in gastric biopsies are identified, an intervention carried out and a second biopsy evaluated to test the lack of progression on the regression of specific markers. The first phases of this approach should provide information on the relevance and responsiveness of the markers, hopefully identifying those which could be tested in large numbers in trials aimed at reduction of cancer rates.

## CONCLUSIONS

The evidence at hand suggests strongly that the gastric precancerous process involves a gradual loss of cell differentiation. The final product is a neoplastic cell which expresses phenotypes of different gastric and intestinal cells somewhat reminiscent of multipotential cells found in the glandular necks. The aetiological factors influencing this process appear to act in different stages of the process. Irritants such as sodium chloride induce atrophy and facilitate the action of mutagens in the induction of dysplasia. Nitrite, a presumed mutagen precursor, induces metaplasia and dysplasia. Beta-carotene acts at the late stages of the chain inhibiting dysplasia and carcinoma.

Several markers of loss of differentiation are available, and there is a need to identify which markers are relevant in order to design intervention strategies.

ACKNOWLEDGEMENT

The work was supported by Program Project Grant PO1-CA-28842 from the National Cancer Institute, National Institutes of Health, Bethesda, MD.

REFERENCES

1.  Bara J, Hamelin L, Martin E, Burtin P (1981) Int J Cancer 28:711-719

2.  Chen V, Abu-Elyazeed R, Zavala D. The use of urinary sodium to creatine ration as an index of salt intake in case-control studies. Submitted for publication

3.  Ciclitira PJ, Macartney JC, Evan G (1987) Journal of Pathology 151:293-296

4.  Cordon-Cardo C, Lloyd KO, Sakamoto J, McGroarty ME, Old LJ Melamed MR (1986) Int J Cancer 37:667-676

5.  Correa P (1988) Am J Gastroenterology. In press

6.  Correa P (1983) Cancer Surveys 2:437-450

7.  Correa P, Fontham ET, Pickle LW, Chen VW, Lin Y, Haenszel W (1985) JNCI 75:645-654

8.  Cuello C, Correa P, Zarama G, Lopex J, Murray J, Godillo A (1979) Am J Surg Path 3:491-500

9.  DeBoer WG, Forsyth A, Nairn RC (1969) Br Med J 3: 93-94

10. Filipe MI (1988) In Reed PI, Hill MJ (eds) Gastric Carcinogenesis. Elsevier, Amsterdam, pp

11. Fontham E, Zavala D, Correa P, Rodriguez E, Hunter F, Haenszel W, Tannenbaum SR (1986) J Natl Cancr Inst 76:621-627

12. Haenszel W, Correa P, Lopez A, Cuello C, Zarama G, Zavala D, Fontham E (1985) Int J Cancer 36:43-48

13. Higgins PJ, Correa P, Cuello C, Lipkin M (1984) Oncology 41:73-76

14. Jass JR (1983) Histopathology 7:181-193

15. Kato Y, Kitagawa T, Sugano H, Karatsuka H (1986) 14th Intl Cancer Congress. Abstract 2288

16. Kodama M, Hiroshi Y, Ishidate T, Kamiyama S, Masuda H, Stemmermann GN, Heilbrun LK, Hankin JH (1982) J Natl Cancer Inst 68:401-405

17  Kroposki H, Stepleski Z, Mitchell K, Herlyn M (1979) Som Cell Genet 5:957-972.

18. Lee P, Mori T, Fujimoto N, Nakamura T, Masuzawa M, Kosaki G (1979) In: Lehmann FG (ed) Carcino-Embryonic Proteins Elsevier/North-Holland Biomedical Press, Amsterdam, Vol II, pp373-378

19. Lipkin M, Correa P, Mikol IB, Higgins PJ, Cuello C, Zarama G, Fontham E, Zavala D (1985) J Natl Cancer Inst 75:613-619

20. Marshall B (1986) J Inf Dis 153:650-657

21. Matsukura N, Kawachi T, Sugimura T, Ohnuki T, Higo M, Itabashi M, Hirota T, Kitaoka H (1980) Acta Histochem Cytochem 13:499-507

22. Matsukura N, Suzuki K, Kawachi T, Aoyagi M, Sugimura T, Kitaoka H, Numajiri H, Shirota A, Itabashi M, Hirota T (1980) J Natl Cancer Inst 65:231-240

23. Ming SC, Goldman H, Freiman DG (1967) Cancer 20:1418-1429

24. Mollicone R, Bara J, LePendu J, Oriol R (1985) Lab Invest 53:219-227.

25. Montes G, Cuello C, Correa P (1985) J Cancer Res Clin Oncol 109:42-45

26. Munoz N, Matko I (1972) Cancer Res 39:99-105

27. Nardewelli J, Bara J, Rosa B, Burtin P (1983) J Histochem Cytochem 31:366-375.

28. Nardelli J, Loridon-Rosa B, Bara J, Burtin P (1984) Cancer Research 44:4157-4163

29. Nitt D, Farini R, Grassi F, Cardin F, DiMario F, Piccoli A, Vianello F, Farinati F, Favrettie F, Lise M, Naccarato R (1983) Cancer 52:2334-2337

30. Noguchi M, Hirohashi S, Shimosato Y, Thor A, Schlom J, Tsunokawa Y, Terada M, Sugimura T (1980) J Natl Cancer Inst 77:379-385

31. Nomura A, Stemmermann GN, Samloff M (1980) Am Int Med 93:537-540

32. Santamaria L, Bianchi A, Ravetto C, Arnaboldi A, Santogati G, Andreoni L (1987) J Nutr Growth and Cancer 4:175-181

33. Sipponen P, Liudgren J (1986) Acta Path Immunol Scand 94:305-311

34. Sipponen P, Seppala K, Varis K, Hjelt L, Ihamaki T, Kekki M, Siurala M (1980) Acta Path Microbiol Scand 88:217-224

35. Skinner JM, Whitehead R (1982) Europ J Cancer 18:227-235

36. Stemmermann GN, Samloff IM, Hayashi T (1985) Appl Pathol 3:159-163

37. Tatematsu M, Takahashi M, Fukushima S, Hananouchi M, Shirai T (1975) J Natl Cancer Inst 55:101-106

38. Wakabayashi K, Nagao M, Ochiai M, Fujita Y, Tahira T, Nakayasu M, Ohgaki H, Takayama S, Sugimura T (1987) In: Bartsch H, O'Neill I, Schulte-Hermann R, (eds) Relevance of N-Nitroso Compounds to Human Cancer: Exposures and Mechanisms. Oxford University Press, Oxford, Vol 84, pp287-291

39. Weissburger JH, Margvardt H, Hirota N, Mori H, Williams GM (1980) J Natl Cancer Inst 64:163-167

40. Yang D, Tannenbaum SR, Buchi G, Lee GCM (1984) Carcinogenesis 5:1219-1224

© Elsevier Science Publishers B.V. (Biomedical Division)
Gastric carcinogenesis. P.I. Reed, M.J. Hill, editors.

CAMPYLOBACTER PYLORI AND PRECANCEROUS LESIONS

BARRIE RATHBONE AND JUDITH WYATT
Departments of Medicine and Pathology, St Jame's University Hospital, Leeds LS9
7TF, UK

INTRODUCTION

The study of gastric carcinogenesis has been based on data from two main sources: from epidemiological studies relating to genetic and environmental factors, and from histological changes associated with carcinoma. These have led to the hypothesis that chronic gastritis is an initial and common precursor lesion on which metaplastic and dysplastic changes may occur and culminate in carcinomatous change.

Non-autoimmune chronic gastritis has been assumed to be the end result of repeated insults to the gastric mucosa, by factors such as alcohol, smoking, hot drinks and reflux of duodenal contents. There are few data however to substantiate these aetiological factors. Isolation of a Gram-negative microaerophilic organism was first reported in 1983 from the gastric mucosa of patients with chronic gastritis (25,41). This organism was originally called a camplylobacter-like organism, then Campylobacter pyloridis and is now known as Campylobacter pylori.

The association between C. pylori and gastric carcinoma has yet to be formally investigated, but the increasing evidence implicating this newly identified bacterium with the pathogenesis of chronic gastritis warrants its inclusion in the symposium.

C. PYLORI - BACKGROUND

While observations of spiral bacteria colonizing gastric mucosa in man and animals date back to the turn of the century (5,8,19), the human organism has only recently been isolated and characterised (26). Although colonizing gastritic mucosa in large numbers, the bacteria are difficult to see on H&E stained sections and therefore have until recently been generally overlooked. The bacteria are easily demonstrated by a number of histological stains including Warthin-Starry (41), modified Giemsa (11) and acridine orange (40) and their strong association with gastric inflammation has now been confirmed worldwide (38).

The C. pylori cultured from gastric biopsies are Gram-negative, spiral, flagellated organisms which grow under microaerophilic conditions. Biochemically the bacteria are interesting, having a marked urease activity (20) which enables colonisation to be diagnosed by a gastric biopsy urease test (24) or a urea breath test (10). In vitro the organisms are sensitive to a wide range of antibacterial agents including bismuth compounds (22). Immunologically the organisms stimulate a local

138

(42) and systemic immune response (17,29,35) the latter being an additional method of diagnosing colonisation.

The reported prevalence of C. pylori in chronic gastritis varies rom 60 to 100% and in non-gastritics from 0-20% (38). This range probably reflects differences in terminology and methodology, as well as geographic variaiton. In our experience, C. pylori are visible histologically in 90% patients with chronic gastritis, and in no patients where the gastric mucosa (antrum and body) is entirely normal. C. pylori are commonly present in patients with gastric ulceration (about 70%) and even more prevalent in duodenal ulceration (95%).

Colonisation by C. pylori appears to be a chronic infection, which once acquired usually persists for years and perhaps for life. The bacterium has only ever been isolated from gastric type epithelium in the stomach, oesophagus or duodenum and its environmental source and usual mode of transmission are unknown. It is common in the apparently normal general population, where its prevalence increases with age; in the UK from 10% in young adults to 50% in the elderly (16). This age-related increase in prevalence closely mirrors that of chronic gastritis, and reports from different areas are suggesting a geographic variation in the prevalence of C. pylori which may match that recognised for chronic gastritis. In high prevalence areas (Africa, Peru), C. pylori is commonly acquired in childhood, whereas this is rare in Europe and North America (6).

## C. PYLORI AND CHRONIC GASTRITIS

Characteristically, gastric mucosa colonized by C. pylori shows chronic inflammatory changes which are more severe in the antrum than the body, or may be limited to the antrum (41). There is an increase in the number of plasma cells, lymphocytes, and histiocytes in the lamina propria, a lengthening of the gastric foveoli, and commonly an active gastritis with intra-epithelial neutrophils present usually at the base of the gastric pits. C. pylori is equally common in superficial and atrophic gastritis; foci of intestinal metaplasia are not colonized by the bacteria, but it is usually present on the adjacent gastric type epithelium in active atrophic gastritis. Lymphoid follicles are often seen in C. pylori-associated gastritis, and are a specific feature of that condition. These follicles are particularly marked in colonized children and are often visible endoscopically.

The histology of C. pylori-associated gastritis is consistent with both the 'hypersecretory' and 'environmental' patterns of gastritis described by Correa (2) although in our experience the inflammation is never patchy in the gastric antrum. However, in those cases of C. pylori-negative gastritis, there is commonly a different pattern of inflammation, (44) either a predominantly body gastritis as in autoimmune gastritis, or features of bile reflux, or rarely a pattern of 'lymphocytic' gastritis (4).

The specific association of C. pylori with 'type B' non-autoimmune gastritis implies that it is not simply a commensal organism in an already inflamed stomach. Other evidence supporting a causal role comes from ingestion and treatment studies. Two volunteers have ingested live C. pylori and in both cases the previously normal gastric mucosa became colonized and inflamed. In one case, the gastritis and bacterial colonisation was acute and self-limiting (27) while in the second chronic colonisation occurred, the acute gastritis became chronic and the subject became seropositive (28).

Small outbreaks of transmissible gastritis have occasionally been recognised (28,33). Retrospective analysis of biopsy material demonstrated that these subjects had C. pylori associated gastritis, but no pre-outbreak biopsies were available. Recent serological studies on stored serum from cases in one of these outbreaks have demonstrated the development of a C. pylori specific antibody response in affected individuals.

A large number of small treatment studies have been attempted with differing agents and have demonstrated that in vitro sensitivity is a poor guide to in vivo activity. The most useful agents have been bismuth compounds (23) (long used for dyspepsia as well as ulcer healing) and amoxycillin (1). Clearance of the organism from the stomach is associated with an improvement in gastritis. Relapse of infection is however a common problem, and this is accompanied by a return of the inflammation (39).

Local immunological and animal studies also provide circumstantial evidence supporting a causal role for C. pylori in chronic gastritis. In colonized patients at least part of the local immune response is directed against C. pylori antigens (36). Specific local immunoglobulins are produced and active inflammation is associated with coating of the bacteria by opsonising antibodies (42). C pylori also induces inflammation in certain susceptible animal models (eg gnotobiotic piglets (18)), and a naturally acquired gastritis in monkeys is associated with colonisation by a closely related if not identical organism (30).

Precisely how C. pylori may cause inflammation has not yet been fully elucidated. This is a non-invasive bacterium, which inhabits a zone on the surface of the gastric epithelium and the deeper levels of the covering mucus gel where the pH is near neutral. The organism is visible, usually in great numbers, particularly at epithelial cell junctions. C. pylori exhibits certain properties which are highly adapted to this environment - brisk motility in viscous media, strong urease activity allowing it to withstand a reduction in pH, attachment to gastric epithelial cells, microaerophilia - enabling it to live where (to our knowledge) no other bacteria are present. It appears likely that a degree of inflammation is beneficial to C. pylori, by increasing the transudate of nutrients across the epithelium (12). Several mechanisms by which such inflammation may be induced have been suggested, (see Rathbone and Wyatt (39) for a summary) although at present these are largely hypothetical proposals.

There is some evidence of toxin production by C. pylori, with certain strains producing culture supernatant which are cytopathic to cell lines. Ammonia produced by the bacterial urease may also be damaging. There is also evidence that C. pylori has mucolytic enzymes which might impair the integrity of the mucus-bicarbonate barrier. Like enteropathogenic E. coli, C. pylori forms adhesion pedistals, which may in some way directly damage the cell. Whatever the mechanism of damage it is clear that the presence of C. pylori is strongly immunogenic, and that in some way the bacterium eludes the host's attempts to clear it. The result is a sustained equilibrium in which the integrity of the epithelium is compromised by virtue of the continued, low grade inflammation.

## C. PYLORI ASSOCIATION WITH PRECANCEROUS CONDITIONS
### Intestinal Metaplasia

Focal areas of intestinal metaplasia are often present in patients with campylobacter-associated gastritis. The metaplastic epithelium is not itself colonized by the bacteria, but providing gastric type epithelium is sufficiently represented in the biopsies, the prevalence of C. pylori appears to be the same in chronic gastritis with and without intestinal metaplasia. This specificity for gastric epithelium is also apparent in the duodenum, where C. pylori is observed only in association with gastric metaplasia (43).

Whether this sparing of intestinal epithelium by C. pylori also encompasses type II, incomplete metaplasia is unclear. It is our impression that colonisation of such eptihelium does occasionally occur, in patients in whom there is heavy colonisaiton of non-metaplastic gastric epithelium.

Areas of dysplasia seen on biopsy are not usually colonized by C. pylori, although again the bacteria may be present on adjacent inflamed epithelium. Similarly, the surface of a gastric carcinoma does not show colonisation.

### Autoimmune Chronic Gastritis

The prevalence of C. pylori in patients with pernicious anaemia is significantly lower than that in type B chronic gastritis (7,31,34) and also lower than in the age matched 'normal' population. This observation has been reported by sveral groups, and cannot be explained simply on the basis of sampling error due to inclusion of itnestinal metaplasia in the biopsies. The low prevalence of C. pylori in these patients with gastric inflammation has ben cited in support of C. pylori having a causative role in antral gastritis, rather than it being a simple opportunist colonizing already inflamed gastric mucosa. C. pylori is not therefore implicated as a factor in the small proportion of gastric carcinomas that arise as a complication of pernicious anaemia.

## Partial Gastrectomy

Although the incidence of gastric carcinoma in gastric stumps years after partial gastrectomy is debated, most authorities consider that previous gastric surgery confers an increased risk of gastric neoplasia.

The gastric mucosa in the operated stomach shows a characteristic appearance of faveolar hyperplasia and oedema which correlates with the degree of bile reflux present, so called 'reflux gastritis' (3). C. pylori are infrequently associated with histological reflux gastritis. Patients treated surgically for duodenal ulcer with partial gastrectomy or gastroenterostomy frequently develop typical reflux gastritis, associated with an absence of C. pylori (32). Since the prevalence of C. pylori in active duodenal ulcer is of the order of 95%, this implies that the development of reflux gastritis promotes eradication of the bacteria, perhaps because of the bile sensitivity of the organism. Thus it was proposed that following partial gastrectomy the pattern of gastritis changed from a campylobacter-associated antral gastritis to campylobacter-negative reflux gastritis .

## Menetriers Disease

Menetrier's disease, a condition characterised histologically by gross faveolar hyperplasia with lengthening and cystic dilatation of gastric pits, and associated clinically with protein loss from the gastric mucosa, is a rare disease of unknown cause. This is another condition where C. pylori has recently been proposed as a possible aetiological agent (21). A self limiting protein losing gastropathy in children has also been linked with C. pylori (13), but much further work is needed before the importance of these bacteria in Menetrier's disease is clarified.

## Gastric Carcinoma

It is well recognised that most patients with gastric cancer have chronic gastritis in the non-neoplastic gastric mucosa, usually of the type and distribution which is associated with C. pylori colonisation. However, reports on the prevalence of C. pylori in patients with gastric cancer have been slow to emerge (14). This is in part because retrospective studies based on the morphology of the bacteria in histological sections are less reliable in this situation, for several reasons. Firstly, routine biopsies from patients with gastric cancer may not include sufficient non-neoplastic mucosa. Secondly, a mixed gastric flora is commonly present in patients with an ulcerating gastric tumour; this may include bacteria with similar morphology to C. pylori. Finally, the bacteria are difficult to recognise in surgical resection specimens, perhaps because fixation is delayed relative to that of endoscopic gastric biopsies. Bearing in mind these limitations the prevalence of C.

pylori in a series of biopsies from gastric cancer patients is shown in Table 1. Forty-six per cent of the 52 patients with adequate gastric mucosa were C. pylori positive. These cases showed a strong association with activity of the gastritis, and were independent of the presence of intestinal metaplasia. Prospective studies are clearly needed to clarify the relationship between C. pylori and the presence of gastric carcinoma.

TABLE 1

C. PYLORI IN NON-NEOPLASTIC GASTRIC BIOPSIES FROM PATIENTS WITH GASTRIC CARCINOMA: RELATIONSHIP TO CHRONIC GASTRITIS

|  | C. pylori +ve (24) | C. pylori -ve (28) |
|---|---|---|
| Active chronic gastritis | 17 | 2 |
| Inactive chronic gastritis | 5 | 13 |
| Quiescent chronic gastritis | 2 | 5 |
| Reflux gastritis | 0 | 6 |
| Normal histology | 0 | 2 |
| Intestinal metaplasia: | | |
| present | 10 | 16 |
| absent | 13 | 15 |

C. pylori are not nitrate-reducing and hence will not directly promote nitroso compound formation. However as the severity of the gastritis increases and there is atrophy of gastric glands and a consequent hypochlorhydria, colonisation of the stomach by nitrate-reducing bacteria will occur.

Another factor which may be relevant is gastric juice ascorbic acid. In healthy subjects ascorbic acid appears concentrated in gastric juice compared to serum, recent studies have shown however that in C. pylori-associated chronic gastritis the concentrations are reduced and in the biologically inactive form (15). Whether this is related directly to the bacteria or the epithelial inflammation is unclear.

CONCLUSIONS

The recently discovered organism C. pylori is strongly implicated in the aetiology of non-autoimmune chronic gastritis. It can also act as a marker (using serology or urea breath test) by which chronic gastritis can be studied epidemiologically without the need to resort to endoscopy.

To date there is no direct evidence linking C. pylori to gastric carcinoma. C. pylori is associated with chronic gastritis, and chronic gastritis is associated with the development of neoplasia. Chronic gastritis is a state of increased epithelial cell turnover in the gastric mucosa, and as such fulfills the criteria for a promotional effect in association with other initiating factors. If C. pylori is to be inserted into a model of carcinogenesis, then this would be at an early stage in the events culminating in neoplasia.

△ Much work is still required to clarify the exact role of C. pylori in gastric inflammation, and the association of campylobacter-associated gastritis with gastric carcinoma has yet to be properly investigated. However its importance as a newly recognised causal agent in chronic gastritis must invite speculation on C. pylori as a potentially reversible factor in the early stages of gastric carcinogenesis.

△ Clearly much work is required to elucidate the exact role of C. pylori in gastric inflammation. As well as being exciting in terms of its possible aetiological role it also raises the possibility of treating or preventing the precancerous lesion chronic gastritis in populations at high risk.

## REFERENCES

1. Burette A, Glupczynski Y, Dereuk M, Labbe M, Deltenre M (1988) In: Campylobacter IV: Proceddings of the IVth International workshop on Campylobacter Infections. In press

2. Correa P (1980) Front Gastrointest Res 6:98-108

3. Dixon MF, O'Connor HJ, Axon ATR, King RFJG, Johnston D (1986) J Clin pathol 39:524-30

4. Dixon MF, Wyatt JI, Burke DA, Rathbone BJ (1988) J Pathol 154:125-32

5. Doenges JL (1939) Arch Pathol 27:469-477

6. Drumm B, Sherman P, Cutz E, Karmali M (1987) NEJM 316:1557-61.

7. Flegjou PF, Bahame B, Smith A, Stockbrugger RW, Rhode J, Price AB (1988) J Pathol 154:86A

8. Freedburg AS, Barron LE (1940) Am J Dig Dis 7:443-445

9. Gledhill T, Leicester RJ, Addis B et al (1985) Br Med J 290:1383-6

10. Graham DY, Klein PD, Evans DG, et al (1986) Gastroenterol 90:1435

11. Gray SF, Wyatt JI, Rathbone BJ (1986) J Clin Pathol 39:1279-1280

12. Hazell SL, Lee A, Brady L, Hennessy W (1986) J Infect Dis 153:658-663

13. Hill ID, Sinclair-Smith C, Lastovica AJ, Bowie MD, Emms M (1987) Arch Dis Children 62:1215-1219

14. Jiang SJ, Liu WZ, Zhang DZ et al (1987) Scand J Gastroenterol 22:553-8

15. Johnson AW, Rathbone BJ, Kelleher J, Heatley RV, Losowsky MS (1986) 70 (suppl 13):38P

16. Jones DM, Eldridge J, Fox AJ, Sethi P, Whorwell PJ (1986) J Med Microbiol 22:57-62

17. Kaldor J, Tee W, McCarthy P, Watson J, Dwyer B (1985) Lancet i:921

18. Krakowka S, Morgan DR, Kraft WG, Leunk Rd (1987) Infect and Immun

144

55:2789-2796

19.  Krienitz W (1906) Dtsh Med Wochenschr 22:872

20.  Langenberg M-L, Tytgat GNJ, Schipper MEJ, Rietra PJGM, Zanen HC (1984) Lancet i:1348

21.  Lepore MJ, Smith FB, Bonanno CA (1988) Lancet i:466

22.  McNulty CAM, Dent J, Wise R (1985) Antimicrob Agents Chemother 28:837-838

23.  McNulty CAM, Gearty JC, Crump B et al (1986) Br Med J 293:645-9

24.  McNulty CAM, wise R (1985) Lancet i:1443-1444

25.  Marshall BJ (1983) Lancet i:1273-1275

26.  Marshall BJ (1984) Lancet i:1311-1315

27.  Marshall BJ, Armstrong JA, McGechie DB, Glancy RJ (1985) Med J Australia 142:436-9

28.  Morris A, Nicholson G (1987) Am J Gastro 82:192-199

29.  Newell DG (1987) Serodiagnosis and Immunotherapy 1:204-217

30.  Newell DG, Baskerville A (1988) In: Campylobacter IV: Proceedings of the IVth International Workshop on Campylobacter Infections. In Press

31.  O'Connor HJ, Axon ATR, Dixon MF (1984) Lancet ii:1091

32.  O'Connor HJ, Dixon MF, Wyat JI et al (1986) Lancet ii:1178-81

33.  Ramsay EJ, Carey KV, Peterson WL et al (1979) Gastroenterology 76:1449-57

34.  Rathbone BJ, Shires SE, Townsend C et al (1988) In: Campylobacter IV: Proceedings of the IVth International Workshop on Campylobacter Infections. In Press

35.  Rathbone BJ, Wyatt JI, Worsley BW (1986) Gut 27:642-647

36.  Wyatt JI, Rathbone BJ (1988) Scand J Gastro Suppl. In Press

37.  Rathbone BJ, Wyatt JI (1988) Scand J Gastroenterol Suppl.In Press

38.  Rathbone BJ, Wyatt JI, Heatley RV (1988) In: Eds Rees WDW. MTP Press, in press

39.  Rauws EA, Langenberg W, Houthoff HJ, Zanen HC, Tytgat GNJ (1988) Gastroenterol 94:33-40

40.  Walters LL, Budin RE, Paull G (1986) Lancet i:42

41.  Warren JR (1983) Lancet i:1273

42.  Wyatt JI, Rathbone BJ, Heatley RV (1986) J Clin Pathol 39:863-870

43.  Wyatt JI, Rathbone BJ, Dixon MF, Heatley RV (1987) J Clin Pathol 40:841-8

44.  Wyatt JI, Dixon MF (1988) J Pathol 154:113-124

# GASTRIC LUMINAL FACTORS

GASTROINTESTINAL FACTORS

© Elsevier Science Publishers B.V. (Biomedical Division)
Gastric carcinogenesis. P.I. Reed, M.J. Hill, editors.

ENDOGENOUS NITROSAMINE FORMATION AND NITRATE BURDEN IN
RELATION TO GASTRIC CANCER EPIDEMIOLOGY

ROLF PREUSSMANN AND ANTHONY R TRICKER

Institute for Chemotherapy and Toxicology, German Cancer Research Centre, Im
Neuenheimer Feld 280, D-6900 Heidelberg, Federal Republic of Germany

INTRODUCTION

Gastric cancer can be histologically subdivided into two main types; the so called
intestinal and diffuse types (36).    Both types of cancer have characteristic
predisposing and precursor pathological states. Atrophic gastritis and intestinal
metaplasia occur as precursor lesions to intestinal type cancer whilst gastric
atrophy is not strongly associated with diffuse type cancers which normally occur in
areas of otherwise healthy mucosa.  In the latter type, environmental factors appear
not to be very significant whilst intestinal type cancers are associated with high
nitrate and salt exposures and poor nutritional status.   Hypochlorhydria has been
reported in 85-90% of gastric cancer patients (25).  Hypochlorhydria resulting from
pernicious anaemia or following Polya gastrectomy has been associated with an
increased incidence of gastric cancer (intestinal type) and in both cases is
considered to be a precancerous condition.  This led Correa et al (8) to propose a
postulated aetiopathology of intestinal type gastric cancer via a multi-stage
sequence of events. Initiation of this sequence is due to the loss of gastric acid and
to the development of gastric atrophy.  Under these conditions a resident bacterial
flora of nitrate reducing bacteria occurs whose metabolic products (eg N-nitroso
compounds) induce atrophic gastritis followed by intestinal metaplasia with
increasing severity of epithelial dysplasia and eventually cancer.  However, the
endogenous formation of N-nitrosamines is not confined to the Correa hypothesis,
since nitrosation also occurs under normal gastric conditions (55).   N-nitroso
compounds, which may be formed in vivo by either chemical nitrosation with
bacterially formed nitrite or by the bacteria themselves, have been shown to be
carcinogenic in all mammalian species tested (49).

Over the last decade, several epidemiological studies have made correlations
between nitrate exposure and cancer risk.  However, recent work has taken a
contradicatory stand against the previous hypothesis that a high exogenous nitrate
exposure increases the risk of cancer (primarily gastric cancer).   The most
important short-term health effect of high nitrate burden is methaemoglobinaemia
in infants (77) and the suggested development of neural tube defects (12) in babies
whose mothers were exposed to high levels of nitrates in drinking water.  A long-
term high exogenous exposure to nitrate may well result in an increased risk of

cancer in some populations, however several other factors related to both nitrate exposure and endogenous nitrosamine formation have to be taken into consideration before cancer risk can be correlated to nitrate exposure. These factors include the way in which nitrate burden is calculated, the significance of endogenous nitrate synthesis, the role of dietary or endogenous amines and their potential endogenous nitrosation via chemical interaction, bacteria or stimulated macrophages. All of which may be further influenced by abnormal pathological conditions in the population under investigation. Occasional, exceptionally high exposures to nitrate also present an increased risk, particularly with respect to the short-term increase in the availability of gastric nitrate and nitrite for endogenous nitrosation reactions.

Epidemiological studies often fail to take these factors into consideration, this may account for some of the conflicting epidemiological results relating nitrate exposure to gastric cancer risk which are discussed in the following chapter.

CHEMISTRY OF NITROSATION

The major source of gastric juice nitrite is the bacterial reduction of nitrate which occurs primarily in the oral cavity but also in the stomach. Under the acidic conditions normally prevailing in the stomach, nitrite has a very short half-life so that gastric nitrite concentrations are usually very low. However, in the neutral stomach nitrite is very much more stable giving rise to higher nitrite concentrations in gastric juice. There is a clear relationship between gastric nitrite concentration and the risk of intestinal metaplasia and epithelial dysplasia in the atrophic stomach. Gastric juice nitrite concentrations have been shown to correlate with the severity of dysplasia in several studies; however there is no evidence to show that nitrite per se causes dysplasia or that it is toxic to the gastric mucosa. Thus the effect must be due to the production of a toxic or carcinogenic metabolite; the action of nitrite as a substrate for carcinogenic N-nitroso compound formation has been suggested (52). Experimental animals fed with secondary amines and high nitrite concentrations show tumor induction typical for the corresponding N-nitroso compounds (54). The endogenous formation of N-nitroso compounds in the human stomach has been demonstrated following the introduction of the "N-nitrosoproline-Test" (47).

For secondary amines, the rate of nitrosation follows second order reaction kinetics as shown in Figure 1. At low concentrations of nitrite, the potential for endogenous nitrosamine formation is relatively small but as the nitrite concentraton increases a disporportionate increase in nitrosation occurs. However, at any given nitrite concentration, the rate of formation of N-nitrosamides may exceed that of N-nitrosamines (41) and this may be more significant at low nitrite concentrations. N-nitrosamides are direct acting carcinogens which unlike N-nitrosamines do not require metabolic activation and therefore produce local as well as systemic tumors. The presence of catalysts such as chloride, iodide, thiocyanate and thiourea (39) changes the kinetics so that amine nitrosation becomes proportional only to the nitrite concentration.

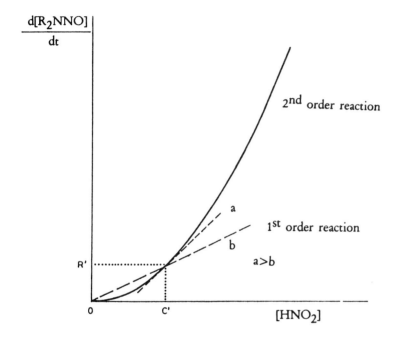

Fig. 1. Rate of nitrosation for secondary amines.

In the upper intestinal tract, salivary nitrate and nitrite are reabsorbed into the blood stream where nitrite reacts immediately with haemoglobin to yield nitrosohaemoglobin. Nitrate remains in circulation and is partially excreted via the kidney (65-70%), faeces (3-10%) or re-enters the oral cavity via the salivary glands. Approximately 25% of exogenous nitrate is taken up from the circulation by the salivary ducts (58) and the amount of nitrate in human saliva ranges from 200 to 600 uM (21). However, significantly higher concentrations may be found after intake of nitrate rich vegetables (58) or in people with poor oral hygiene. Re-introduction of nitrate into the oral cavity results in increased nitrite exposure via bacterial reduction of nitrate with a maximum salivary nitrite concentration occuring 1-2

TABLE 1
DAILY DIETARY BURDEN OF NITRATE AND NITRITE

| Country | Period (years) | Method of Determination | Intake (mg/person/day) | | | | Reference |
|---|---|---|---|---|---|---|---|
| | | | Nitrate Mean | (Range) | Nitrite Mean | (Range | |
| Sweden | - | 24 hour diet analysis | 49 | (26-81) | 3.8 | (0.6-7.4) | 32 |
| FRG | 1971-73 | Combined methods | 75 | (55-95) | 3.3 | 2.5-3.9) | 57 |
| Switzerland | 1977 | Consumer statistics | 91 | - | - | - | 66 |
| Netherlands | 1976-78 | Combined methods | 98 | - | 6.7 | - | 69 |
| | 1976-78 | 24 hour diet analysis | 110 | (9-706) | 2.8 | (0-40.5) | 60 |
| USA | 1971-73 | Consumer statistics | 106 | - | 2.6 | - | 76 |
| UK | 1970-71 | Consumer statistics | 116 | - | - | - | 71 |
| | - | Consumer statistics | 119 | - | - | - | 18 |
| Serbia | 1972-74 | 24 hour diet analyis | 113 | (12-321) | 0.8 | (0.3-5.1) | 1 |
| | 1977-78 | 24 hour diet analysis | 114 | (34-318) | 11 | (0.7-33) | 1 |
| Czechoslovakia | - | Consumer statistics | 142 | - | - | - | 68 |
| Singapore | 1982 | Combined methods | 250 | - | - | - | 14 |
| Japan | 1977 | 24 hour diet analysis | 218 | (44-864) | 0.4 | (0-1.3) | 29 |
| | 1977 | 24 hour diet analysis | 295 | (97-677) | - | - | 38 |
| | 1972-74 | Consumer statistics | 314 | - | 1.2 | - | 30 |
| | 1974 | Consumer statistics | 286 | - | 0.6 | - | 30 |
| | 1976 | Consumer statistics | 245 | - | 1.3 | - | 30 |

hours after consumption of nitrate and nitrite containing foodstuffs as well as restarting the circulation of both nitrate and nitrite. This process has been summarised in Figure 2.

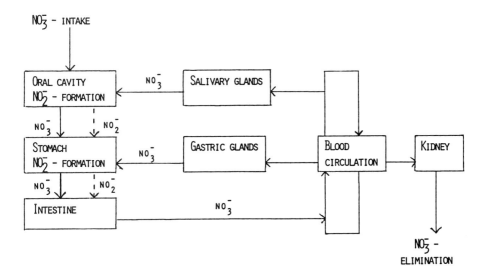

Fig. 2. Flow diagram of gastrointestinal nitrate circulation.

Dietary nitrate and nitrite burden calculated by consumer statistics from per capita daily consumption based on gross retained imports and/or direct analysis of duplicate 24-hour diets is summarized in Table 1.

In addition to the dietary exposure to nitrate and nitrite, recent research has shown that endogenous formation of both nitrate and nitrite from organic precursors may occur under certain pathological conditions. Mammals maintained on low nitrate diets show a higher urinary excretion of nitrate than that which can be obtained from the diet indicating that nitrate synthesis occurs endogenously at a basal rate. In rats, this basal rate of nitrate synthesis can be increased 10-fold after stimulation of the immune system induced by treatment with Escherichia coli lipopolysaccharide (E. coli LPS) (70). In vitro studies using primary murine macrophage cultures stimulated with E. coli LPS and lymphokines such as gamma-interferon, synthesis of both nitrate and nitrite has been demonstrated (62,63).

Further studies have shown that stimulated macrophage cultures nitrosate secondary amines via an active intermediate formed during nitrite synthesis (44) in which L-arginine acts as a specific precursor to both nitrate and nitrite (31). Therefore, endogenous nitrate and nitrosamine formation may be highly significant in pathological conditions involving inflammatory diseases.

## ENDOGENOUS NITROSATION IN HUMANS

The endogenous formation of N-nitroso compounds has been demonstrated to occur in humans (55,47,17). Under normal conditions, the in vivo formation of N-nitrosodimethylamine (NDMA) cannot be directly monitored in urine due to its high metabolic conversion rate (>99.9%) in the liver. Partial inhibition of NDMA metabolism by the consumption of ethanol has been used to study the in vivo nitrosation of amidopyrine, an easily nitrosatable precursor to NDMA by urinary monitoring of NDMA excretion following simultaneous consumption of ethanol and amidopyrine (59).

The effect of dietary nitrate burden on endogenous nitrosamine formation has been shown by increasing the dietary nitrate burden from 75 mg/day(57) to 675 mg/day resulting in a 10 fold increase in the urinary excretion of endogenously formed N-nitrosamino acids in a human volunteer (67).

Pathological conditions causing a decrease in gastric acidity which may occur in patients who have pernicious anaemia (53), have undergone Billroth I or Billroth II operations (56) or have received long-term treatment with $H_2$-receptor antagonists such as cimetidine and ranitidine (16,50) may result in changes in the gastric bacterial flora allowing a bacterial overgrowth of denitrifying bacteria which may produce a large increase in the availability of nitrite for reaction with nitrosatable species. Whilst the availability of nitrite is increased, the pH conditions are unfavourable for the chemical nitrosation of most secondary amino compounds (51). Application of the "NPRO-Test" in pernicious anaemia patients with decreased gastric acidity shows weak evidence for a second gastric pH maxima occurring at pH 5.5-6.0 for proline nitrosation in addition to the expected classical acid mediated nitrosation maxima at pH 2.5 (22). Leach et al (37) have shown that denitrifying bacteria (eg P. aeruginosa, Neisseria spp., Alcaligenes faecalis, Bacillus licheniformis) present in achlorhydric gastric juice can increase the rate of nitrosation of secondary amines by two to three orders of magnitude under in vitro conditions not suitable for chemical nitrosation. Under the same conditions, actively nitrosating non-nitrifying bacteria would be expected to form nitrosamines in the achlorhydric stomach at rates of 10 to 100-fold in excess of acid mediated nitrosation.

EPIDEMIOLOGY

Epidemiological reports on the correlations of high incidences or risks of human cancer with nitrate burden have been a contentious area of research for nearly a decade. One major point which is seldom emphasised is that nitrate per se does not present a cancer risk, however it acts as a precursor to nitrite (via bacterial reduction) which reacts either directly or indirectly (again via bacteria) to produce N-nitroso compounds which are known potent carcinogens in experimental animals. These tests provide potential evidence for the carcinogenicity of N-nitroso compounds in man. As a result, nitrate burden should be regarded as an "indirect risk" factor and N-nitroso compound formation as a "direct risk" factor in human carcinogenesis. The latter has been correlated to gastric cancer risk via "indirect risk" estimation based on nitrate burden. The results for selected epidemiological studies correlating nitrate exposure as well as the major source of dietary nitrate against gastric cancer risk are summarized in Table 2. In the Colombian study (10) it was reported that gastric cancer risk correlated with urinary nitrate excretion but not with salivary nitrate. Thus, although a high nitrate burden could be shown (determined in urine) in this area of high gastric cancer incidence, the nitrate burden (as determined in saliva) did not correlate with the levels of gastric cancer. In a later study (4) higher levels of nitrate in the urine of school children from a low risk area of gastric cancer in Chile was reported. In an area of low gastric cancer risk in Iran (15) very high levels of salivary nitrate in children were also reported. Both studies clearly disagree with the hypothesis correlating nitrate intake directly against gastric cancer as reported by Hartman (23). However, according to Mirvish (42) the data used in the last study was sufficient to support the conclusion that "nitrate intake correlated against gastric cancer mortalities in 12 countries".

154

TABLE 2

THE CORRELATION BETWEEN HIGH NITRATE BURDEN AND GASTRIC CANCER RISK

| Country | High nitrite source | Correlation | Reference |
|---|---|---|---|
| Chile | Vegetables and drinking water due to high use of nitrate fertilizer | Positive | 44 |
| | | Positive | 45 |
| | | Positive | 46 |
| | | Negative | 47 |
| | | Negative | 48 |
| China | Vegetables due to low molybdenum content of soil. Drinking water | Positive | 49 |
| Columbia | Vegetables and drinking water due to high nitrate content of soil | Positive | 50 |
| Denmark | Drinking water | Positive[+] | 52 |
| England | Drinking water | Negative | 52 |
| | | Negative | 53 |
| | | Negative | 27 |
| | | Inconsistent | 54 |
| | | Inconsistent | 55 |
| Hungary | Drinking water | Inconsistent | 56 |
| Italy | Drinking water | Positive[+] | 57 |
| Japan | Vegetables due to high nitrate content of soil | Negative | 58 |

+Both studies present limited data for comparison of high and low risk populations, results should be regarded as inconsistent.

More recent results suggest that nitrate may be inversely related to gastric cancer risk, whether nitrate is measured in drinking water (6) or in saliva (18). The results of both studies have been suggested to be questionable and should be reviewed cautiously (43,48). The importance of dietary factors, particularly vegetables, has been raised in two epidemiological studies: In preliminary data from China the nitrate and nitrite burden from vegetables and drinking water was shown to be higher in high risk areas for gastric cancer, similarly these areas showed increased levels of nitrate and nitrite in saliva and gastric juice of fasting patients with chronic gastritis (78). In Japan, nitrate burden determined by urinary excreton was higher in the low risk area as compared to the high risk area for gastric cancer and correlated well with the consumption of vegetables (35). Thus it appears that the diet and dietary souce of nitrate may be more significant than the total nitrate burden. The latter may be particularly relevant in situations in which occasional very high exposures to dietary nitrate occur. The occurrence of nitrosation inhibitors (vitamin C and phenolic compounds) which also occur in vegetables and reduce the risk of cancer by endogenous N-nitrosamine formation (43,64) in low risk populations which show high nitrate levels in saliva (18).

Recent epidemiological studies on dietary nitrate and its involvement in the aetiology of gastric cancer have been critically reviewed (19). In developed countries only weak evidence for dietary nitrate involvement in gastric cancer exists; nitrate burden and exposure in drinking water is increasing whilst at the same time stomach cancer is declining. In some developing countries (eg Colombia and China) a more complex situation occurs in which low gastric acidity and dietary deficiencies are prevalent and a high nitrate burden may be one of several factors responsible for the increase of gastric cancer in these populations.

The results from epidemiological studies relating nitrate burden to gastric cancer risk, in particular negative studies, can also be interpreted as showing that amine precursors to N-nitroso compounds (and alkylating species) relevant to the induction of human gastric cancer are not ubiquitous in the human diet or gastric juice.

AMINE PRECURSORS

Whilst it is possible to determine simple volatile and non-volatile N-nitroso compounds in the human diet, our lack of knowledge on specific amine precursors to potentially relevant gastric carcinogens (after reaction with nitrite) remains a central problem in our understanding of human gastric carcinogenesis. Positive epidemiological studies in developing countries have often emphasised nutritional status and specific dietary items in association with gastric cancer risk (20). However, no single dietary item has been found which could explain the worldwide differences in gastric cancer risk. For example, smoked fish has been positively associated with gastric cancer risk in Iceland (13), Japan (26) and Norway (7) but is uncommon in Colombia (9).

Following nitrosation, fish commonly used in the Japanese diet has been shown to induce adenocarcinoma of the glandular stomach in experimental rats (75). Sun-dried herrings and sardines show mutagenic activity (5500-12400 revertants/g, respectively) after nitrite treatment (72).

Epidemiological data from Colombia (9) has shown a high intake of fava beans (Vicia faba) in high risk populations for gastric cancer. Nitrosated fava beans produce a very potent mutagen whose precursor was identified (Fig. 3) as 4-chloro-6-methoxyindole (79). Indole-3-acetonitrile, 4-methoxyindole-3-acetonitrile and 4-methoxyindole-3-aldehyde have also been identified as nitrosatable mutagen precursors in Chinese cabbage (73), following nitrite treatment all three compounds were shown to be direct-acting mutagens in TA98 and TA100. Indole-3-acetonitrile reacts rapidly with physiologically feasible concentrations of nitrite to produce the N-1-nitroso analogue, the latter causes DNA modifications in the glandular stomach of rats following incubation. This obsrvation suggests that substituted indoles in the diet which are widely abundant in green plants of the brassica family could also react with nitrite in the human stomach resulting in DNA damage.

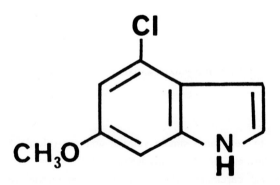

Fig. 3. 4 chloro-6-methoxy indole (present in fava beans)

Tyramine (45) and substituted beta-carbolines; (-)-(1S,3S)-1-methyl-1,2,3,4-

tetrahydro-beta-carboline-3-carboxylic acid ((-)-(1S,3S)-MTCA) and its stereo-isomer (-)-(1R,3S)-MTCA formed by the condensation of L-tryptophan and acetaldehyde (77) have been identified as nitrosatable mutagen precursors in soya sauce. Nitrite treatment of tyramine yields 3-diazotyramine which has been shown to be carcinogenic in rats producing squamous cell carcinomas in the oral cavity. A similar diazonium compound, 4-(hydroxymethyl)-benzenediazonium ion, formed from agaritine in mushrooms has been reported to induce glandular stomach tumors in mice (65).

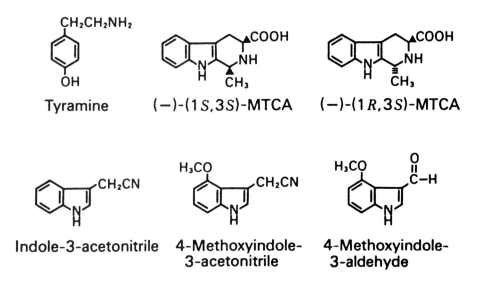

Tyramine          (−)-(1S,3S)-MTCA          (−)-(1R,3S)-MTCA

Indole-3-acetonitrile     4-Methoxyindole-     4-Methoxyindole-
                            3-acetonitrile          3-aldehyde

Fig. 4. Structures of mutagenic precursors isolated from soya sauce (top row) and Chinese cabbage (bottom row)

Pyrolysis (dry heating) of food products rich in amino acids and proteins produces highly mutagenic nitrosatable 3-ring N-heterocyclic aromatic amine compounds. Japanese foods: broiled dried fish, grilled beef, chicken and onions have been shown to contain between 1-650 ug/kg pyrolysis products (28). The most important representatives of this group of compounds have been shown to be carcinogenic in a number of animal species, 2-amino-3-methylimidazo(4,5-f)quinoline (IQ) and 2-

amino-3,4-dimethylimidazo(4,5-f)quinoline (MeIQ) show carcinogenic activity in mice producing predominantly liver, but also forestomach and lung tumors (46). Pyrolysis products are both potent mutagens and animal carcinogens per se, following nitrosation aminoimidazoquinoline (IQ and MeIQ) and aminomethylimidazoquinoxalines retain their mutagenic potential, other classes of pyrolysis products show reduced or no mutagenic activity.

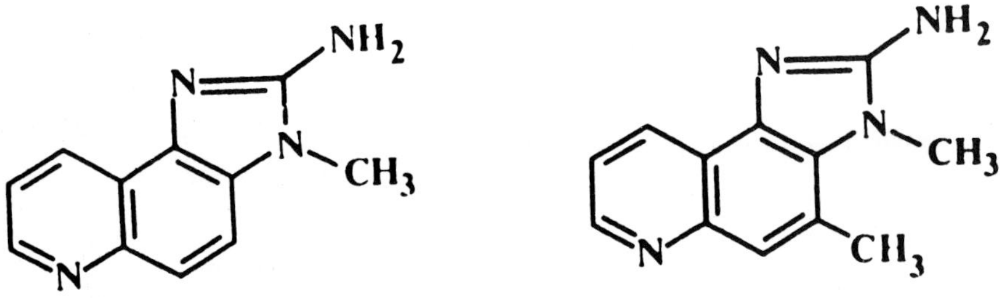

**IQ**                    **MeIQ**

Fig. 5. Pyrolysis products inducing forestomach tumors in mice.

The previously mentioned examples (shown in Figures 3,4 and 5) illustrate some examples of rather complex species which may in specific cases be involved in the aetiology of human gastric carcinogenesis. Relatively simple primary amines which occur naturally in all foodstuffs could present a more significant risk factor in the aetiology of human carcinogenesis. Nitrosation of primary amines under in vivo conditions produces a diazonium cation which breaks down rapidly under physiological conditions to yield a carbonium ion with a very short half-life. The in vivo nitrosation of $^{14}$C-labelled methylamine with nitrite in rats produced 7-($^{14}$C)methylguanine in DNA isolated from the gastrointestinal tract (27), thus indicating that carbonium ions (alkylating agents) formed by the nitrosation of primary amines have a sufficiently long half-life and are stable enough to penetrate cell membranes. The resultant formation of carbonium ions near to the epithelial mucosa via the interaction of nitrite with primary amines could under specific conditions initiate a cellular DNA modification.

In vitro studies (40) show that the formation of N-nitrosodialkyamines from the nitrosation of primary amines seems negligible in most cases in comparison to the direct alkylation of biological macromolecules or other nucleophiles by the intermediate cabonium ion formed on nitrosation of primary amines.

CONCLUSIONS

Despite the many complex interactions involved in the endogenous formation of N-nitroso compounds, particularly with regard to the participation of bacteria and simulated macrophages under abnormal pathological conditions, it still remains valid that nitrate burden plays a significant role in human carcinogenesis. However, it must be emphasised that the role of nitrosatable amine precursors, and in particular primary amines, whether obtained through dietary sources or endogenously formed (as bacterial metabolites) and their availability in the human stomach is equally, if not more important, than the nitrate burden. In the presence of nitrosatable amine precursors, the potential formation of N-nitroso compounds and/or alkylating species which may be relevant to the induction fo gastric cancer and other human cancers remains a plausable working hypothesis. The occurrence and nature of nitrosatable amines in the human stomach remains as one of the most important missing links in our knowledge about endogenous nitrosamine formation.

Whilst no systematic studies on the availability of nitrosatable amines in the human stomach are available and detailed knowledge of specific amine precursors in the diet are lacking, endogenous formation of N-nitroso compounds from secondary amines and the formation of carbonium ions (direct alkylating species) from primary amines as a risk factor for human carcinogenesis remains a valid working hypothesis.

REFERENCES

1. Adamovic VM, Hus M (1979) Hrana Ishrana 20:35-40

2. Amadori D, Ravaioli A, Gardini A, Liverani M, Zoli W, Tonelli B, Ridolfi R, Gentilini P (1980) Tumori 66:145-152

3. Armijo R, Coulson AH (1975) Int J epidemiol 4:301-309

4. Armijo R, Gonzalez A, Orellana M, Coulson AH, Sayre JW, Detels R (1981) Int J Epidemiol 10:57-211

5. Beresford SA (1981) Int J Epidemiol 10:103-115

6. Beresford SA (1985) Int J Epidemiol 14:57-63

7. Bjelke E (1974) Scand J Gastroenterol 9 (Supp 31):1-253

8.  Correa P, Haenszel W, Cuello C (1975) Lancet i:58-60

9.  Correa P, Cuello C, Fajardo LF (1983) J Natl Cancer Inst 70:673-678

10. Cuello C, Correa P, Haenszel W, Gordillo G, Brown C, Archer M, Tannenbaum S (1976) J Natl Cancer Inst 57:1015-10201

11. Davies JM (1980) Br J Cancer 41:438-445

12. Dorsch MM, Scragg RKR, McMichael AJ, Baghurst PA, Dyer KF (1984) Am J Epidemiol 119:473-486

13. Dungal N (1961) JAMA 178:789-798

14. Dutt MC, Lim HY, Chew RKH (1987) Fd Chem Toxic 25:515-520

15. Eisenbrand G, Spiegelhalder B, Preussmann R (1980) Oncology 37:227-231

16. Elder JB, Ganguli PC, Gillespie IE (1979) Lancet i:1005-1006

17. Fine DH, Ross R, Rounbehler DP, Silvergleid A, Song L (1977) Nature 265:753-755

18. Forman D, Al-Dabbagh S, Doll R (1985) Nautre 313:620-625

19. Fraser P, Chivers C (1981) Sci Total Environ 18:103-116

20. Fraser P (1985) In: Interpretation of Negative Epidemiological Evidence for Carcinogenicity. (IARC Sci Publ No 65) International Agency for Research on Cancer, Lyon pp183-194

21. Geboers J, Joossens JV, Kesteloot H (1985) In: Joossens JV, Hill MJ, Geboers J (eds) Diet and Human Carcinogenesis. Elsevier Scientific Publishers B.V. pp81-95

22. Green LC, Wagner DA, Glogowski J, Skipper PL, Wishnok JS, Tannenbaum SR (1982) Analyt Biochem 126:131-138

23. Hall CN, Kirkham JS, Northfield TC (1987) Gut 28:216-220

24. Hartman PE (1983) Environ Mutagen 5:111-121

25. Hill MJ, Hawksworth G, Tattersall G (1973) Br J Cancer 28:562-567

26. Hitchcock DR, Scheiner SL (1965) Surg Gynecol Obstet 113:665-672

27. Hirayama T (1975) Cancer Res 35:3460-3463

28. Huber KW, Lutz WK (1984) Carcinogenesis 5:1729-1732

29. IARC (1983) Some Food Additives IARC Monographs, Vol 31, Lyon pp36-38

30. Ishiwata H, Mizushiro H, Tanimura A, Murata T (1978) J Food Hyg Soc Japan 19:318-322

31. Ishiwata H, Tanimura A (1982) J Hyg Chem (Japan) 28:171-183

32. Iyengar R, Stuehr DJ, Marletta MA (1987) Proc Natl Acad Sci USA 84:6369-6373

33. Jagerstad M, Norden A, Nilsson R (1977) Ambio 6:276-277

34. Jensen OM (1982) Ecotoxicol Environ Saf 6:258-267

35. Juhasz L, Hill MJ, Nagy G (1980) In: Walker EA, Castegnaro M, Griciute L, Borzsonyi M (eds) N-nitroso Compounds: Analysis, Formation and Occurrence. (IARC Sci Publ No 31). International Agency for Research on Cancer, Lyon. pp619-623

36. Kamiyama S, Ohshima H, Shimada A, Saito N, Bourgada M-C, Ziegler P, Bartsch H (1987) In: Bartsch H, O'Neill I, Schulte-Hermann R (eds) The Relevance of N-nitroso Compounds to Human Cancer: Exposure and

Mechanisms. (IARC Sci Publ No 84). International Agency for Research on Cancer, Lyon. pp497-502

37. Lauren P (1965) Acta Path Microbiol Scand 64:31-49

38. Leach SA, Thompson M, Hill M (1987) Carcinogenesis 8:1907-1912

39. Maruyama S, Shimizu S, Muramatsu K (1979) J Food Hyg Soc Japan 20:276-281

40. Masui M, Fugisawa H, Ohmori H (1982) Chem Pharm Bull (Tokyo) 30:593-597

41. Mende P, Unpublished results

42. Mirvish SS (1975) Toxicol Appl Pharmacol 31:325-351

43. Mirvish SS (1983) J Natl Cancer Inst 71:631-647

44. Mirvish SS (1985) Nature 315:461-462

45. Miwa M, Stuehr DJ, Marletta MA, Wishnok JS, Tannenbaum SR (1987) Carcinogenesis 8:955-958

46. Ochiai M, Wakabayashi K, Nagao M, Sugimura T (1984) Gann 75:1-3

47. Ohgaki H, Matsukura N, Morino K, Kawachi T, Sugimura T, Takayama S (1984) Carcinogenesis 5:815-819

48. Ohshima H, Bartsch H (1981) Cancer Res 41:3658-3662

49. Pocock SJ (1985) Hum Toxicol 4:471-477

50. Preussmann R, Stewart BW (1984) ACS Monograph Series, No 182 pp643-828

51. Reed PI, Cassell PG, Walters CL (1979) Lancet i:1234-1235

52. Ruddell WSJ (1981) Lancet i:784-785

53. Ruddell WSJ, Bone ES, Hill MJ, Walters CL (1976) Lancet ii:1037-1039

54. Ruddell WSJ, Bone ES, Hill MJ, Walters CL (1978) Lancet i:521-523

55. Sander J, Burkle G 91969) Z Krebsforsch 76:93-96

56. Sander J, Schweinsburg F, Menz HP (1968) Z Physiol Chem 349:1691-1697

57. Schlag P, Bockler R, Ulrich H, Peter M, Merkle P, Herfarth C (1980) Lancet i:727-729

58. Selenka F, Brand-Grimm D (1976) Zbl Bakt Hyg I Abt, Orig B 162:449-466

59. Spiegelhalder B, Eisenbrand G, Preussmann R (1976) Food Cosmet Toxicol 14:545-548

60. Spiegelhalder B, Preussmann R (1985) Carcinogenesis 6:545-548

61. Stephany RW, Shuller PL (1980) Oncology 37:203-210

62. Stuehr DJ, Marletta MA (1985) Proc Natl Acad Sci USA 82:773807742

63. Stuehr DJ, Marletta MA (1987) J Immunol 139:518-525

64. Tannenbaum SR, Correa P (1985) Nature 317:675-676

65. Toth B, Nagel D, Ross A (1982) Br J Cancer 46:417-422

66. Tremp E (1980) Mitt Gebiete Lebensm Hyg 71:182-194

67. Tricker AR, Preussmann R (1987) Cancer Letters 34:39-47

68. Turek B, Hlavsova D, Tucek J, Waldman J, Cerna J (1980) In: Walker EA, Griciute L, Castegnaro M, Borzsonyi M (eds) N-nitroso Compounds: Analysis, Formation and Occurrence. (IARC Sci Publ No 31). International Agency for Research on Cancer, Lyon, pp625-632

69. Vos RH de, Dokkum W van (1980) Centraal Institut voor Voedingsonderzoek

TNO, CIVO-Ziest. Rapport nr R6331

70. Wagner DA, Young VR, Tannenbaum SR (1983) Proc Natl Acad Sci USA 80:4518-4521

71. Walker R (1975) J Sci Fd Agric 26:1735-1738

72. Wakabayashi K, Nagao M, Chung TH, Yin M, Karai I, Ochiai M, Tahira T, Sugimura T (1985) Mutat Res 158:119-124

73. Wakabayashi K, Nagao M, Tahira T, Yamaizumi Z, Katayama M, Marumo S, Sugimura T (1986) Mutagenesis 1:423-426

74. Wakabayashi K, Ochiai M, Saito H, Tsuda M, Suwa Y, Nagao M, Sugimura T (1983) Proc Natl Acad Sci USA 80:2912-2916

75. Weisburger JH, Marquardt H, Hirota H, Mori N, Williams GM (1980) J Natl Cancer Inst 64:163-167

76. White Jr JW (1975,1976) J Agric Food Chem 23:886-891; 24:202

77. World Health Organisation (1984) Health Hazards from Nitrate in Drinking Water. Copenhagen

78. Xu G-W (1981) J R Soc Med 74:210-211

79. Yang D, Tannenbaum SR, Bucki B, Lee GCM (1984) Carcinogenesis 5:1219-1224

80. Zaldivar R (1977) Experimentia 33:264-265

81. Zaldivar R, Wetterstrand WH (1975) Experimentia 31:1354-1355

82. Zaldivar R, Robinson H (1973) Z Krebsforsch 80:289-295

© *Elsevier Science Publishers B.V. (Biomedical Division)*
*Gastric carcinogenesis. P.I. Reed, M.J. Hill, editors.*

GASTRIC JUICE N-NITROSO COMPOUNDS

C L WALTERS

Department of Biochemistry, University of Surrey, Guildford, Surrey GU2 5XH, UK

INTRODUCTION

N-nitroso compounds, and particularly the N-nitrosamides and -guanidines, have been found to induce tumours in the glandular stomachs of experimental animals. Fasting gastric juices contain both nitrosating and amino or amido precursors to N-nitroso compounds. The great majority of such compounds formed on deliberate nitrosation are not simple volatile N-nitrosamines but are more complex in character. Some ingested foods will contribute nitrite and preformed N-nitroso compounds to the gastric milieu and most will introduce nitrosable amines, amides, etc. Thus, a considerable number of N-nitroso compounds could be formed in situ, the limiting factor being the low level of nitrite in the normal acidic stomach, which is supplemented by that formed in the saliva from dietary nitrate.

Since it would be impracticable to estimate each of so many N-nitroso compounds individually, it has been necessary to determine gastric concentrations as a group and to differentiate them from nitrite and as many other types of compounds derived from it as possible. A number of modifications of the original method of Walters et al (27) have been employed, all reliant upon the determination of nitric oxide from its chemiluminescent response after reaction with ozone.

Hypochlorhydria often precedes and/or accompanies gastric cancer and this is associated with colonization of the stomach with bacteria, including those capable of reducing nitrate, which is distributed widely throughout biological materials. Thus, any increase in gastric N-nitroso compounds resulting from such an increase in pH would represent a risk factor in the development of cancer in this organ. Whilst there is universal agreement that the concentration of the precursor, nitrite, correlates with the pH of the gastric juice controversy remains as to whether an increase in pH is accompanied by a rise in the level of N-nitroso compounds as a group.

PRECURSORS TO N-NITROSO COMPOUNDS IN GASTRIC JUICE

Nitrite

Nitrate ingested in vegetables, water supplies, etc, is absorbed into the blood stream from which a part at least is secreted by the salivary glands into the mouth. Subsequently a proportion of that secreted is reduced by nitrate-reducing bacteria and possibly mammalian enzyme systems to provide a backgorund level of nitrite in the saliva on a normal diet of the order of 100 uM (25). The consumption of meals containing nitrate rich foods results in a rise in the salivary nitrite concentration within 1-2 hours to values approaching 2 mM (28). Other workers have observed succeeding peaks of salivary nitrite as the swallowed nitrite is recirculated through the blood stream (23).

Following the consumption of a meal including foods prepared with nitrite itself the concentration of this additive increased rapidly in the stomach to a maximum of about 0.3 mM and subsequently started to decline approximately 50 minutes after the meal as the pH began to fall towards its fasting value (28).

Nitrite reacts readily with phenols, amines, thiols, etc, at the pH of the normal fasting stomach and thus its background concentration is low under these conditions, with a mean level of 1.7 $\pm$ 0.3 uM for pH values of less than 2.5. This value was raised to a mean of 30.4 $\pm$ 4.9 uM in gastric juices with a pH exceeding 5.0 (20).

Amino and Related Compounds

The nonprotein nitrogen content of normal gastric juice was reported by Martin as long ago as 1931 (12) to range from 0.20-0.48 g/l, equivalent to a concentration of 14-34 mmol/l for compounds containing one nitrogen atom. The corresponding ranges for achlorhydric gastric juice and that in pernicious anaemia (PA) were 0.30-0.90 g and 0.60-1.5 g nonprotein nitrogen/l. Many non-nitrosatable amino acids and other compounds would be included, of course, in these totals. Later, a comparison was made between the amino acid composition of pooled normal human gastric juice and that from PA patients (6). The concentrations of all amino acids quoted were increased in the PA samples by factors ranging from 1.4-13.5. As a potentially nitrosatable amino acid, the mean concentrations of arginine in normal and PA gastric juices were 13 mg/l (90 umol/l) and 47 mg/l (330 umol/l) respectively. For proline, the corresponding figures wre 3.0 and 13 mg/l (26 and 110 umol/l respectively).

A number of comparisons have been made between the levels of amino acids in normal gastric juice and those from persons suffering from pernicious anaemia (6). Three out of four studies recorded three to five times the levels of total or individual amino acids in this pathological condition, which is associated wtih an elevated incidence of gastric cancer. Nevertheless, the reduced volume of fasting gastric juice present in the stomach in pernicious anaemia must also be considered in comparing the availability of nitrosatable precursors.

N-nitroso compounds can be derived from not only secondary amines, amides, guanidines, etc, but also from tertiary amines and presumably amides by nitrosative cleavage. It is most realistic, therefore, to determine nitrosatable precursors as N-nitroso compounds after deliberate nitrosation under optimal conditions. After treatment of pooled acidic gastric juice with a high concentration of nitrous acid at pH 2.0 in the presence of thiocyanate as a catalyst only very small quantities of simple volatile N-nitrosamines were formed (29). The main compounds of this type detected by gas chromatographhy with the Thermal Energy Analyser as a highly selective detector were N-nitrosodimethylamine (NDMA) and -pyrrolidine (NPyr) at concentrations approximating to 0.05 and 0.005 umol/l respectively. After methylation with diazomethane, about 40% of the total response of the nitrosated gastric components to the group selective procedure of Walters et al (27) could be separated by gas chromatographhy with a Thermal Energy Analyser as detector. This fraction includes the N-nitroso derivatives of proline, hydroxyproline, sarcosine, thiazolidine and oxazolidine. According to Outram and Pollock (15), the treatment of dipeptides with nitrous acid results in an intramolecular reaction with the formation of N-nitrosated dialkanoic acids. Under standardized conditions, the yields of N-nitroso compounds as a group ranged from 0.09% for alanylhistidine to almost 13% for alanylmethionine, assuming the introduction of one N-nitroso group per molecule. Similarly, the extent of nitrosation of glycylphenylalanine (1.5%) was much less than that of phenylalanylglycine (8.3%).

Bile reflux has been associated with an increased incidence of gastric cancer observed in the stump following some types of partial gastrectomy. Comparisons have been made between the precursors to N-nitroso compounds available in bulked samples of pentagastrin-stimulated (A) and bile-contaminated (B) gastric juice. Overall, type B has been found to contain more than four times as much precursor to N-nitroso compounds. Around 5% of the response of B was in the form of precursors to N-nitrosodimethylamine (NDMA) and -pyrrolidine (NPyr) as compared with the very low yield from A. Similarly, the amounts of precursors which can be converted by methylation into a form(s) amenable to gas chromatography were more than ten times greater in the bile contaminated juice than in A. The mean content of nitrosatable amines in 85 samples of acidic gastric juice was 0.165 mM, in considerable excess of the normal nitrite concentration.

## CATALYSTS AND INHIBITORS OF NITROSATION

Apart from the chloride anion, the principal catalyst relevant to the stomach is thiocyanate, which can stimulate the rate of formation of N-nitrosamines at low pH values by up to several hundred fold. Thiocyanate is present in almost all gastric juices, and particularly in that of smokers, at potentially catalytic levels (26).

Ascorbic acid, which inhibits the reaction of secondary amines with nitrous acid, is ingested in foods. Gastric juices also contain phenols, which scavenge nitrite from its reactions to form N-nitroso compounds. However, the products of the reactions of some phenols with nitrite can stimulate the conversion of secondary amines into their N-nitroso derivatives (16).

## DETERMINATION OF N-NITROSO COMPOUNDS

Since gastric juices contain nitrite which could give rise to N-nitroso compounds as artifacts it has been necessary to remove this contaminant before the determination of such carcinogens in these fluids. Of the reagents employed for this purpose, most researchers have made use of sulphamic acid, which lowers the pH of the gastric juice to 1-2 and rapidly scavenges the nitrite present. An attempt was made by Bavin, Darkin and Viney (1) to remove nitrite from gastric juices at a pH of 4.0 at which the stability of N-nitrosamides is maximal. To this end, they added hydrazine sulphate and then buffered the gastric juice at the desired pH. According to Pignatelli et al (17), however, the depletion of nitrite occurred at the lower pH of <2 directly after the addition of hydrazine sulphate. In some cases, moreover, and notably that of N-methyl-N'-nitro-N-nitrosoguanidine (MNNG), stability during storage at -20°C was markedly better using sulphamic acid than hydrazine sulphate.

All procedures for the determination of N-nitroso compounds as a group have made use of chemiluminescence analysers designed for the assay of nitric oxide as activated nitrogen dioxide following reaction with ozone. With one exception, all have employed hydrogen bromide as a denitrosating agent.

In the method of Walters et al (27), extracts of gastric juices are injected into refluxing ethyl acetate under an atmosphere of nitrogen. After any evolution of nitric oxide from heat labile compounds has ceased, acetic acid is injected to decompose any nitrite which might have escaped the action of the scavenger of choice. Hydrogen bromide in acetic acid is then injected to liberate nitric oxide from any N-nitroso compounds present. The subsequent injection of an authentic N-nitroso compound provides a standardized evolution of nitric oxide on which to base the calculation of their total concentration in the gastric juice.

In order to accelerate the above procedure, Bavin et al (1) proposed a modification in which the gastric juices themselves, after treatment with hydrazine sulphate to remove nitrite are injected into hydrogen bromide in refluxing ethyl acetate under nitrogen. The nitric oxide evolved is considered to emanate from N-nitroso compounds present. However, it was pointed out by Smith, Walters and Reed (22) that this fraction would include nitric oxide arising from other compounds derived from nitrite in a biological system, such as the S-nitrosothiols. This fact has also been considered by Pignatelli et al (17) in their modified procedure for the analysis of total N-nitroso compounds in gastric juice. After treatment of the juices with sulphamic acid to remove nitrite, each was analysed by two separate procedures. In the first, an aliquot was injected directly into refluxing ethyl acetate containing acetic acid with the addition of 0.1% hydrochloric acid; the nitric oxide evolved was derived from any compounds such as the S-nitrosothiols, labile under these conditions, which did not lead to the decomposition of N-nitroso compounds.

A second aliquot was injected directly into refluxing ethyl acetate containing hydrogen bromide, the nitric oxide liberated arising from N-nitroso compounds in addition to those labile in acetic acid/hydrochloric acid. By difference, therefore, Pignatelli et al have been able to calculate the concentration of N-nitroso compounds as a group in the gastric juice. At least 50% of samples they examined contained acid-labile compounds which would have been confused for N-nitroso compounds using denitrosation by hydrogen bromide alone throughout the range of pH of the gastric juices with the exception of that from pH 1.6-2.3.

CHEMICAL NITROSATION

The reaction between a secondary amine and nitrite requires both to be in the undissociated form. As the pH is lowered the proportion of nitrite as undissociated nitrous acid becomes greater but the amine is increasingly in the unreactive dissociated form. Thus, the maximum rate of reaction occurs at an optimum pH value in the region of 3.5. The rate of reaction of nitrite with less basic compounds such as the secondary amides continues to increase progressively with fall of pH.

The oxides of nitrogen $N_2O_3$ and $N_2O_4$, which can be obtained readily from nitrite at acid pH under aerobic conditions, are effective nitrosating agents, particularly at an alkaline pH. Nitric oxide, on the other hand, is virtually inactive unless catalysed by, for instance, iodine (3).

BACTERIAL NITROSATION

Evidence has been provided in a number of studies that bacteria can promote the formation of N-nitroso compounds and three possible mechanisms have been proposed (11). Firstly, the action of the bacteria may involve merely the reduction of nitrate to nitrite coupled with acidification of the milieu by the products of bacterial metabolism; both of these processes promote the acid catalysed reactions of nitrite. Secondly, N-nitrosation could be stimulated by products of bacterial secondary metabolism; evidence of such an action was provided by Collins-Thompson et al (4). Finally, the bacterial enzymes themselves could catalyse the N-nitrosation process.

Recently it has been demonstrated (9) that denitrifying bacteria can catalyse N-nitrosation reactions, the rates of reaction being several orders of magnitude greater than those observed with any non-denitrifiers. Nevertheless, potentially relevant bacteria such as E. coli not usually considered to be denitrifiers can also catalyse N-nitrosation reactions but at greatly reduced rates; in fact, bacteria of this latter type probably possess some ability to denitrify in that they produce small amounts of the gaseous oxides of nitrogen when grown anaerobically with nitrate (2). Overall, therefore, it has been shown that some bacteria can promote the process of nitrosation at neutral pH with kinetics consistent with catalysis by enzymes.

## EFFECT OF pH ON LEVELS OF NITRITE IN GASTRIC JUICE

In a study of fasting gastric juices from 69 patients undergoing routine gastrointestinal investigation, Ruddell et al (20) reported an inverse relationship between the nitrite and hydrogen ion concentrations with a highly significant increase in gastric juice nitrite in hypochlorhydric subjects.

Of the 30 patients with no demonstrable gastroduodenal lesions, the gastric juices of 18 had a pH of less than 2.5 and were considered to be normal. The juices of the remaining 12 patients had a pH in excess of 5.0 and comprised the hypochlorhydric normals. The mean nitrite concentration of the normal group, namely 1.7 $\pm$ 0.5 uM (mean - SEM) did not differ significantly from that of the 21 patients with duodenal ulcer in whom its mean concentration was 1.3 $\pm$ 0.3 uM. However, the mean nitrite concentration in the gastic juice of 12 patients with gastric ulcer at a value of 7.9 $\pm$ 4.1 uM was significantly higher (p<0.05) than those for the normal and duodenal ulcer groups which had higher hydrogen ion concentrations. The mean nitrite concentration of the gastric juices of the hypochlorhydric normals (25.6 $\pm$ 3.6 uM) was significantly higher (p<0.05) than those of the other preceeding groups, but did not differ from the value associated with a group of six patients with gastric cancer.

No significant differences between the various diagnostic groups were noted in their levels of thiocyanate, a catalyst of nitrosation at acid pH values, but the concentrations were significantly higher in the juices of 38 smokers in comparison with those of 25 non-smokers. The variations in bacterial counts observed were secondary to those in pH amongst the various groups.

Similar relationships between the nitrite concentration of a gastric juice and its pH have been reported in all similar studies. This is not surprising in the light of the universal availability of nitrate in gastric juices, their colonization with viable nitrate-reducing bacteria at pH value greater than about 5 and the ready reaction of nitrite from the saliva with phenols, amines, thiols, etc, in the stomach at acidic pH values.

## EFFECT OF pH ON LEVELS OF N-NITROSO COMPOUNDS IN GASTRIC JUICE

In a study by Reed et al (18) of sampes of fasting gastric juice from 50 healthy volunteers and 217 patients with common upper gastrointestinal complaints, nitrite was determined before stabilization with sulphamic acid. Using the method of Walters et al (27), the concentration of N-nitroso compounds extractable into ethyl acetate was found to rise in both sexes progressively with age after accounting for the influence of pH. Over the range 18-60 years, the concentration of N-nitroso compounds in normal gastric juices rose from 0.02 to 1.1 uM. For all juices, the rise in concentration from 18-87 years was 0.01 to 40 uM. The pH values of the gastric juices were also found to correlate with age and N-nitroso compounds concentrations were significantly higher in males, taking account of all other factors.

Of greatest importance, however, was the significant relationship observed between pH and the concentration of N-nitroso compounds after allowing for age, sex, smoking, the presence of nitrite and their interactions. Thus the mean level of N-nitroso compounds of 0.10 uM and pH 1.0-1.5 was elevated to 1.2 uM at pH 6.5-9.0. Significant correlations were apparent in several conditions including duodenal ulcer, gastric ulcer, post-vagotomy, pernicious anaemia and gastric cancer. Thus, conditions recognised to be associated with hypochlorhydria such as pernicious anaemia and gastric cancer showed correspondingly higher levels of N-nitroso compounds. Not surprisingly in the circumstances, a highly significant ($p < 0.31 \times 10^{-5}$) relationship was found between bacterial growth and the level of N-nitroso compounds and nitrate reductase-positive organisms were also significantly associated with raised pH ($p < 0.028$).

Similar findings were made by Pignatelli et al (17) in gastric juices from patients before and after operation for duodenal ulcer (n = 59) or with chronic atrophic gastritis (n = 9). The values they obtained for the concentrations of N-nitroso compounds in gastric juices were more in keeping with those reported using the procedure of Walters et al (27) than the elevated levels characteristic of the less selective method of Bavin, Darkin and Viney (1). Their results support the hypothesis that hypochlorhydria permits bacterial overgrowth leading to the increased formation of nitrite and N-nitroso compounds and hence an elevated risk of the development of gastric cancer. So far as the stabilization of gastric juice samples was concerned, Pignatelli et al (17) encountered no formation of N-nitroso compounds as artefacts using sulphamic acid but the use of hydrazine sulphate at pH 4 led to artefactual synthesis in all cases. The stabilities of N-nitroso compounds in the presence of sulphamic acid were often, but not always, greater than those where hydrazine sulphate, buffered to pH 4, had been added.

Of recent years, changes in the pH of gastric juices have occurred as a result of the use of drugs designed to alleviate and/or heal ulcers. It has therefore been of considerable interest to ascertain the effects of such treatments on the concentration of N-nitroso compounds in the stomach. As an example, Sharma et al (21) studied bacterial counts and concentrations of nitrite and N-nitroso compounds in ten healthy volunteers before, during and after treatment with the ATP-ase inhibitor omeprazole. For the latter estimation, the samples of gastric juice were stabilized using sulphamic acid and examined by the procedure of Walters et al (27).

On the 14th and last night of treatment, the mean intragastric acidity had been significantly decreased by 75% (p<0.001). 22 hours after the last dose of omeprazole, there were significant increases in bacterial counts and the concentrations of nitrite and N-nitroso compounds (p<0.001). A fall occurred in the gastric concentration of nitrate, but was not significant. These changes were all resolved three days after discontinuing omeprazole treatment. Similar statistically significant rises in intragastric nitrite and N-nitroso compound concentrations were observed by Stockbrugger et al (24) in 23 patients with duodenal or gastric ulcers treated with the $H_2$ antagonist cimetidine. Reduction of basal acid output by 73% and peak acid output by 36% led to a rise in nitrate reducing bacteria to which the conversion of nitrate to nitrite was closely related.

The method of determination of N-nitroso compounds of Walters et al (27) was also used in a study by Meyrick Thomas et al (13) but the samples of gastric juice were stabilized using hydrazine sulphate in the manner of Bavin, Darkin and Viney (1). In this instance, the gastric contents of 15 persons with peptic ulcer were studied before and on completing six weeks treatment with the $H_2$-blocker ranitidine, twice during maintenance treatment for 9-12 months and one month after stopping the drug. Although intragastric pH, nitrite concentration and counts of total and nitrate-reducing bacteria increased during treatment with the $H_2$ antagonist, there was no significant increase in N-nitroso compounds. In spite of these changes, however, persistent bacterial colonization of the stomach was prevented by an acid tide at some point in each 24 hour study period. One month after stopping one year's treatment with ranitidine all of the variables under study had returned to pretreatment values. Thus, whilst significant positive correlations were observed between pH, nitrite concentration and bacterial counts, the correlations between pH or nitrite concentration and that of N-nitroso compounds as a group were not significant. Chemically, ranitidine acts as a nitrite scavenger, forming a nitrolic acid in the process.

Conflicting results have been reported on the effect of cimetidine on gastric juice N-nitroso compounds. Using the method of determination of Walters et al (27), Reed et al (18) found significantly higher concentrations of N-nitroso compounds and pH levels in 140 patients taking the $H_2$-receptor antagonist in comparison with those in 267 subjects, including 50 healthy volunteers, not taking cimetidine. On the other hand, Milton Thompson et al (14) studied 8 healthy subjects before, during and after cimetidine treatment at hourly or half-hourly intervals for 24 hour periods. No significant differences in intragastric bacterial counts, bacterial species or concentrations of nitrite or N-nitroso compounds were found as a result of this treatment. Both bacterial counts and the nitrite concentration tended to increase with pH but that of N-nitroso concentrations, which were determined by the method of Bavin et al (1) after stabilization with hydrazine sulphate, did not.

Keighley et al (8) also applied the procedure of Bavin et al (1) to the determination of N-nitroso compounds of gastric juices stabilized with hydrazine sulphate. They studied three groups of patients after operations which had cured duodenal ulcers in comparison with a control group. The surgical procedures employed included proximal gastric vagotomy, truncal vagotomy and pyloroplasty. Both counts of nitrate reducing bacteria (p<0.01) and the gastric nitrite concentration (p<0.01) over 24 hours were significantly increased over the controls after truncal vagotomy and antrectomy but no significant difference was observed between the concentrations of N-nitroso compounds in the various groups. Thus, whilst counts of nitrate reducing bacteria and nitrite concentrations increasd with pH those of N-nitroso compounds did not. A similar study was carried out by Hall et al (5) using the same analytical procedures on 9 patients after Polya gastrectomy, 8 with pernicious anaemia and 9 matched controls. Counts of both total and nitrate reducing bacteria (p<0.01) and nitrite concentraions (p<0.01) were positively related to pH whilst those of N-nitroso compounds tended to decrease with increase of pH, ie hypoacidity was not found to enhance nitrosation in these studies.

DISCUSSION

The increase of gastric nitrite concentration with pH reported by all observers to date is in accord with its pattern of stability and the viability of nitrate reducing bacteria. On the other hand, the discrepancies occurring between the various reports of the relationship between the concentration of N-nitroso compounds and pH in gastric juices probably arise from one or more of the variations in the conditions adopted. Thus, the reported formation of N-nitroso compounds as artifacts following the use of hydrazine as a stabilizer could well be responsible for the higher values often reported using this stabilizer. It has been acknowledged that the release of nitric oxide through the action of hydrogen bromide is not entirely restricted to N-nitroso compounds, which can also be derived from nitrolic acids and S-nitrothiols. In addition, the recent studies of Pignatelli et al (17) have confirmed the necessity to take account of other compounds also derived from nitrite in gastric juices which can be confused for N-nitroso compounds when simplified assay procedures are employed.

CONCLUSIONS

The controversy concerning the relationship of the concentration of N-nitroso compounds to pH has not yet been completely resolved. This conclusion will probably have to await the determinations of the individual N-nitroso compounds involved. Nevertheless, Leach, et al (10) have calculated from their own studies that considerably greater concentrations of N-nitrosomorpholine would be formed by bacterial catalysis under conditions relevant to the achlorhydric stomach than would be produced by chemical nitrosation as in the acidic stomach, particularly at very low concentrations of nitrite, such as 3 uM. At the very least, the type of N-nitroso compounds most likely to be formed from precursors available in the gastric juice would include the more complex forms considered to be directly acting carcinogens to the stomach, although even some of the simple volatile N-nitrosamines can act as indirect carcinogens to this organ (7).

## REFERENCES

1. Bavin PMG, Darkin DW, Viney NJ (1982) In: Bartsch H, O'Neill IK, Castegnaro M, Okada M (eds) N-nitroso compounds: Occurrence and Biological Effects, IARC Scientific Publicatons No 41. International Agency for Research on Cancer, Lyon pp337-344

2. Bleakley, BH, Tiedje JM (1982) Appl Environ Microbiol 44:1342-1348

3. Challis BC, Kyrtopoulos SA (1979) J Chem soc Perkin I:299-304

4. Collins-Thompson DL, Sen NP, Aris B, Schwinghamer L (1972) Can J Microbiol 18:1968-1971

5. Hall CN, Darkin DW, Brimblecombe RW, Cook AJ, Kirkham JS, Northfield TC (1986) Gut 86:491-498

6. Heathcote JR, Washington RJ (1965) Nature 207:941-944

7. Homburger F, Handler AH, Soto E, Hsuch SS, Van Dongen CG, Russfield AB (1976) J Natl Cancer Inst 57:141-143

8. Keighley MRB, Younger D, Poxon V, Morris D, Muscroft TJ, Burdon DW, Barnard J, Bavin PMG, Brimblecombe RW, Darkin DW, Moore PJ, Viney NJ (1984) Gut 84:238-245

9. Leach SA, Cook AR, Challis BC, Hill MJ, Thompson MH (1987) In: Bartsch H, O'Neill I, Schulte-Hermann R (eds) The Relevance of N-nitroso compounds to Human Cancer: Exposures and Mechanisms, IARC Scientific Publications No 84. International Agency for Research on Cancer, Lyon pp396-399

10. Leach SA, Thompson M, Hill MJ (1987) Carcinogenesis 8:1907-1912.

11. Leach SA (1988) In: Hill MJ (ed) Nitrosamines: Toxicology and Microbiology, Ellis Horwood, Chichester, in press

12. Martin L (1931) Bull Johns Hopkins Hosp 49:286-301

13. Meyrick Thomas J, Misiewicz JJ, Cook AR, Hill MJ, Smith PLR, Walters CL, Forster JK, Martin LE, Woodings DF (1987) Gut 28:726-738

14. Milton Thompson GJ, Lightfoot NF, Ahmet Z, Hunt RH, Barnard JB, Bavin PMG, Brimblecombe RW, Darkin DW, Moore PJ, Viney NJ (1982) Lancet i:1901-1095

15. Outram JR, Pollock JRA (1984) In: O'Neill IK, Von Borstel RC, Miller CT, Long J, Bartsch H (eds) N-nitroso Compounds: Occurrence, Biological Effects and Relevance to Human Cancer, IARC Scientific Publications No 57. International Agency for Research on Cancer, Lyon pp71-76

16. Pignatelli B, Friesen M, Waler EA (1980) In: Walker EA, Griciute, L, Castegnaro M, Borzsonyi, M (eds) N-nitroso Compounds: Analysis, Formation and Occurrence, IARC Scientific Publications No 31. International Agency for

Research on Cancer, Lyon pp95-106

17. Pignatelli B, Richard I, Bourgade MC, Bartsch H (1987) In: Bartsch H, O'Neill I, Schulte-Hermann R (eds) The Relevance of N-nitroso Compounds to Human Cancer, IARC Scientific Publications No 84. International Agency for Research on Cancer, Lyon pp209-215

18. Reed PI, Smith, PLR, Haines K, House F, Walters CL (1981) Lancet ii:550-552

19. Reed PI, Smith PLR, Haines K, House FR, Walters CL (1981) Lancet ii:553-556

20. Ruddell WSJ, Bone ES, Hill MJ, Blendis LM, Walters CL (1976) Lancet ii:1037-1039

21. Sharma BK, Santana IA, Wood EC, Walt RP, Pereira M, Noone P, Pounder RE, Smith PLR, Walters CL (1984) Brit Med J 289:717-719

22. Smith PLR, Walters CL, Reed PI (1983) Analyst 108:896-898

23. Spiegelhalder B, Eisenbrand G, Preussmann R (1976) Food Cosmet Toxicol 14:545-548

24. Stockbrugger RW, Cotton PB, Eugenides N, Bartholomew BA, Hill MJ, Walters CL (1982) Gut 23:1048-1054

25. Tannenbaum SR, Sinskey M, Weisman D, Bishop W (1974) J Natl Cancer Inst 53:79-83

26. Walters CL, Dyke CS. Saxby MJ, Walker R (1976) In: Walker EA, Bogovski P, Griciute L (eds) Environmental N-nitroso Compounds: Analysis and Formation, IARC Scientific Publications No 14. International Agency for Research on Cancer, Lyon pp181-193

27. Walters CL, Downes MJ, Edwards MW, Smith PLR (1978) Analyst 103:1127-1133

28. Walters CL, Carr FPA, Dyke CS, Saxby MJ, Smith PLR, Walker R (1979) Food Cosmet Toxicol 17:473-479

29. Walters CL, Smith PLR, Reed PI (1982) In: Magee PN (ed) Nitrosamines and Human Cancer, Banbury Report 12. Cold Spring Harbor Laboratory pp445-452

© *Elsevier Science Publishers B.V. (Biomedical Division)*
*Gastric carcinogenesis. P.I. Reed, M.J. Hill, editors.*

# MARKERS FOR INTRAGASTRIC NITROSAMINE FORMATION AND RESULTING DNA DAMAGE

H OHSHIMA, B PIGNATELLLI, C MALAVEILLE, M FRIESEN, S CALMELS, D SHUKER, N MUNOZ AND H BARTSCH

International Agency for Research on Cancer, 150 Cours Albert Thomas 69372, Lyon Cedex 08, France

## INTRODUCTION

Intestinal type stomach cancer, while declining in most populatins in recent years, still remains the most common cancer in both sexes on a worldwide basis (29). This decline in stomach cancer suggests that the majority of cases of this cancer result from environmental causes and, therefore, it could be preventable. Numerous data from several types of epidemiological studies, such as case-control, ecologic, migration and family studies, have revealed various aetiological factors for stomach cancer, including a diet rich in salted or smoked food and low in vitamin C (18). Exposure to nitrate and nitrite, precursors of carcinogenic N-nitroso compounds (NOC), has been also correlated to stomach cancer mortality (24,34). On the other hand, chronic atrophic gastritis (CAG) and intestinal metaplasia (IM) are consistently associated and may represent precancerous conditions of the stomach. In 1975, Correa et al, (10) proposed an aetiological hypothesis linking high rates of stomach cancer with CAG, IM and intragastric NOC formation. They postulated that the hypochlorhydric conditions found in the stomach of patients with CAG and IM may provide a suitable milieu for intragastric formation of NOC owing to the presence of a large number of bacteria, which may be involved in the conversion of nitrate to nitrite and subsequent nitrosation in vivo (8,10,12,36,41,44). NOC are among the most potent chemical carcinogens in laboratory animals, and certain nitrosamides and related carcinogens such as aryldiazonium compounds have been shown to induce glandular stomach adenocarcinomas resembling human gastric cancer (12,41,46). Thus the N-nitrosamides formed in the human stomach through an interaction between nitrite and suitable amino precursors have been suspected of playing an important role in gastric carcinogenesis. However, the questions concerning what kind of NOC are involved and whether the amounts produced in the stomach correlate with the incidence of stomach cancer remain to be answered. During the last few years, several laboratory methods to detect and quantitate the exposure to carcinogens and resulting DNA-damage have been developed. The potential advantages of integrating such methods into epidemiological and clinical studies on stomach cancer are discussed below.

INVESTIGATIVE APPLICATIONS OF THE NPRO TEST

The NPRO Test and Urinary N-nitrosamino acids (NAA) as an Index for Exposure to NOC

Since there have been no reliable methods to estimate the extent of in vivo formaton of NOC in humans, we have developed a non-invasive, simple method for the quantative estimation of endogenous nitrosation (2,3,27). Human urine has been shown to contain several NAA, among which N-nitrosoproline (NPRO), N-nitrosothiazolidine 4-carboxylic acid (NTCA) and N-nitroso 2-methyl thiazolidine 4-carboxylic acid (NMTCA) are the major NAA. Most of these NAA are either non-carcinogenic or weakly carcinogenic and the unchanged compounds are excreted almost quantitatively in the urine of rats after oral administration. For the NPRO test, L-proline, a naturally occurring amino acid, is given to human subjects as a probe for nitrosatable amines. Although NRPO is not carcinogenic in rodents, the mechanism for its formation from proline and nitrosating agents is similar to that for the formation of carcinogenic nitrosamines from other secondary amines. Thus the potential for endogenous nitrosation in human subjects can be quantitated by the amounts of NPRO excreted in the urine after intake of L-proline. Formation in vivo of other nitrosamines could be predicted on the basis of kinetics for nitrosation of secondary amines (28). Based on previous observations that endogenous nitrosation can be blocked to a large extent by ingested ascorbic acid, the difference of the levels of NPRO and other NAA in the urine collected with and without intake of ascorbic acid may reflect endogenous nitrosation.

Urinary Excretion of NAA and Nitrate by Inhibitants in High- and Low-Risk Areas for Stomach Cancer

Exposure to NOC ingested in foods or formed endogenously, was compared in inhabitants in high- and low-risk areas for stomach cancer in northern Japan, by determining urinary levels of NAA as exposure indices (Table 1). Three different samples of 24 hour urine were collected from each of 104 inhabitants of high-risk (Akita) and low-risk (Iwate) areas for stomach cancer according to the following protocols: (a) without ingestion of proline, (b) after ingestion of proline 3-times a day and (c) after ingestion of proline together with vitamin C 3-times a day (19). These samples were analysed for nitrosamino acids, nitrate and chloride ion as indices of the exposure (Table 1). The median values of NPRO and NMTCA excreted in the urine of undosed subjects were not different between the two areas; however, that of NTCA was significantly higher in subjects of the high risk area. After intake of proline, the NPRO level increased significantly only in subjects from the high-risk area, but not in those from the low-risk area; intake of viatmin C inhibited this increase of NPRO and lowered the levels of other nitrosamino acids only in the high-risk subjects. On the contrary, the urinary level of nitrate was higher in subjects of the low-risk area, compared to those of the high-risk area; nitrate levels were found to correlate well with the consumed amounts of vegetables. These results indicate that, although nitrate intake by subjects in the high-risk area is lower, their potential for intragastric nitrosation is higher, suggesting the occurrence of some inhibitory factors for nitrosation in the diet of the low-risk area. Salt intake estimated from the level of chloride ion in the urine did not differ in the two areas.

TABLE 1

MEDIAN (AND 95% CONFIDENCE INTERVALS) FOR VOLUMES OF 24-H URINE AND AMOUNTS OF N-NITROSAMINO ACIDS AND NITRATE DETECTED IN URINE AND P VALUES[a] OF COMPARISON (19)

| Study Area | No of Subjects | N-Nitrosamino Acid (ug/person per day) | | Nitrate[b] (mg/person per day) |
|---|---|---|---|---|
| | | NPRO | Sum[c] | |
| High-risk area (Akita) | | | | |
| Group AA (undosed) | 52 | 3.8 (2.6-5.0) | 20.2 (14.7-26.6) | 95 (73-117) |
| Group AB (proline) | 52 | 12.6 (8.5-16.7) | 43.9 (33.7-54.0) | 116 (83-150) |
| Group AC (proline + vitamin C) | 52 | 3.2 (2.4-4.0) | 15.2 (11.3-19.1) | 130 (107-160) |
| Low-risk area (Iwate) | | | | |
| Group IA (undosed) | 52 | 6.1 (4.1-8.1) | 14.8 (7.4-22.2) | 145 (118-170) |
| Group IB (proline) | 52 | 7.1 (6.6-9.6) | 24.3 19.4-29.2) | 177 (136-219) |
| Group IC (proline + vitamin C) | 52 | 4.9 (3.3-6.5) | 15.8 (9.1-22.4) | 88 (61-115) |
| | | NPRO | Sum | Nitrate |
| AA vs IA | | NS | NS | 0.001 |
| AB vs IB | | 0.001 | 0.001 | NS |
| AC vs IC | | 0.05 | NS | NS |
| AA vs AB | | 0.001 | 0.001 | 0.001 |
| AA vs AC | | NS | 0.01 | 0.005 |
| AB vs AC | | 0.001 | 0.001 | NS |
| IA vs IB | | NS | 0.05 | NS |
| IA vs IC | | NS | NS | NS |
| IB vs IC | | NS | NS | 0.001 |

[a] P values of comparison (NS, Not significant)
[b] Medians (95% confidence intervals) for all Akita subjects and for all Iwate subjects are 116 (104-128) and 140 (117-163) mg/person/day, respectively; difference, $P < 0.07$
[c] Sum of NPRO, NMTCA and NTCA

A study on subjects living in high (rural)- and low (urban)-risk-areas for stomach cancer in Poland has been carried out in collaboration with Dr W Zatonsky, Warsaw, using a similar protocol (NPRO-test, nitrate in urine and dietary questionnaires). A preliminary analysis of the data showed that the results are qualitatively similar to those obtained in the study in Japan.

On the other hand, Chen et al (9), observed no clear correlation between stomach cancer mortality rates and nitrosation potential (as measured by the urinary level of NPRO after the loading dose of proline with and without ascorbic acid) in 26 different rural areas of the People's Republic of China, although there was a moderate, but not significant, tendency for oesophageal cancer mortality rates to be associated positively with nitrosation potential and negatively with background levels of ascorbate in plasma. Similarly, Crespi et al (personal communication) observed no correlation between NPRO levels and incidence of stomach cancer in the subjects with CAG from high risk (San Marino) and low risk (Rome) areas for stomach cancer.

These conflicting results are subject to further studies but may suggest that (i) the above positive results obtained in Japan and Poland may be random findings or (ii) in the case of the latter two negative studies, the majority of human subjects may have already developed CAG and IM, whose gastric pH is not optimal (pH 2) for chemical nitrosation of proline (see below).

Intragastric Nitrosation in Subjects with Precancerous Conditions of the Stomach

The NPRO test has also been applied in a recently completed clinical study to test the hypothesis that subjects with CAG and IM have an elevated nitrosation potential due to the bacterial colonization in the stomach (3,11). The study subjects were selected from those attending the gastroenterology departments of collaborating hospitals. The procedures included completion of a questionnaire, gastroscopy and collection of fasting gastric juice and biopsies. 24-h urine samples were also collected from each subject after the ingestion of 200 ml beetroot juice (containing 260 mg of nitrate) and 30 min later 500 mg L-proline. The subjects fasted for a further 2 hours and avoided foods rich in nitrate and pre-formed NPRO during the period of urine collection. According to the results of the histological evaluation of biopsy samples, the subjects were classified into three groups (I-III): I (n=15), subjects with normal mucosa or with superficial gastritis only; II (n=17), those with mild CAG with or without mild IM; III (n=18), those with moderate and severe CAG with or without IM, and those with dysplasia. The highest yields of NPRO and other NAA (Table 2), after ingestion of loading doses of nitrate and proline, were seen in the subjects with acidic fasting gastric juice (pH 1.5-2). Levels of NPRO were not increased in the subjects with more advanced lesions. However, counts for total and nitrate-reducing bacteria were positively correlated with the pH of gastric juice in these patients.

TABLE 2

URINARY EXCRETION OF N-NITROSAMINO ACIDS IN SUBJECTS WITH NORMAL STOMACH MUCOSA OR WITH SUPERFICIAL GASTRITIS (GROUP I), SUBJECTS WITH MILD CAG, WITH OR WITHOUT MILD IM (GROUP II) AND THOSE WITH MODERATE AND/OR SEVERE CAG WITH OR WITHOUT IM AND THOSE WITH DYSPLASIA (GROUP III) (11)

| Subject Group | No of Subjects | pH of Gastric Juice | N-nitrosamino Acid (ug/person/day) Median (95% confid. interval) | | | |
|---|---|---|---|---|---|---|
| | | | NPRO | NTCA | NMTCA | Sum |
| I | 15 | 1.75 (1.2-8.7) | 14.4 (6.4-17.9) | 6.1 (3.6-9.4) | 1.1 (0.5-4.2) | 27.2 (14.9-36.6) |
| II | 17 | 1.90 (1-7.6) | 12.1 (4.5-20.4) | 4.0 (2.6-7.6) | 2.3 (0.7-6.1) | 24.5 (13.7-34.8) |
| III | 18 | 2.85 (1-7.9) | 6.3 (2.9-9.3) | 3.4 (1.9-4.1) | 1.0 (0.5-2.1) | 13.9 (6.1-i6.1) |

* Significantly different from Groups I and II (P < 0.05)

Similar results have been reported recently by Hall et al (16,17) in patients who had undergone a Billroth II gastrectomy (PG) or had pernicious anaemia (PA), both of which are known to be associated with an increased risk of stomach cancer. Although intragastric levels of bacteria and nitrite were significantly elevated in these patient groups compared to those in healthy matched control subjects, the NPRO levels in urine after doses of nitrate and proline were reduced in the PG and PA patients.

In the two above mentioned studies, the highest yield of NPRO was seen in subjects whose gastric pH was about 1.5-2.0, which coincides with the optimum pH reported for nitrosation of proline in vitro (21). Under such acidic conditions, gastric juice is normally sterile, and, therefore, no correlation was observed between bacterial counts and urinary NPRO level. Thus, these data do not support the notion that the formation of N-nitroso compounds is favoured in the hypoacidic stomach of CAG patients that have an increased bacterial colonization.

Nitrosation in the Achlorhydric Stomach

The findings described above are in contrast to those of other reports that higher levels of bacteria, nitrite and total N-nitroso compounds were detected in the stomach of such patients (36,37,50). The possible reason for this discrepancy could be due to the following:

(1)    The rate for chemical nitrosation of proline under the acidic condition of

the normal stomach may be kinetically much higher than that for the bacterially catalysed nitrosation in the achlorhydric stomach.

(2)    Proline may not be a good substrate for bacterially catalyzed nitrosation. Although bacteria have been shown to catalyse a wide range of secondary amines, the nitrosation activity for proline has been shown to be rather low as compared to that for nitrosation of morpholine (6).

(3)    Only certain types of bacteria, for example, those with a capacity to denitrify (P. aeruginosa, Neisseria spp. etc), may produce greater amounts of NOC in achlorhydric conditions than those formed by acid-catalyzed chemical reaction (7,20).    Thus a small proportion of individuals colonized by bacteria with strong nitrosation activity may produce more NOC and it is conceivable that only those subjects may be at a high risk of developing stomach cancer (21).

(4)    Nitrosation occurring at the border of the normal and metaplastic areas of the stomach may be more important in gastric carcinogenesis than nitrosation in gastric juice.    It hs been postulated that this border could be the most favourable site for chemical nitrosation, because the highest concentration of nitrite is formed by bacteria in the intestinalized areas and the lowest pH is provided by gastric acid secreted by normal mucosa (8).    In fact gastric tumours have been detected frequently in such boundary areas (45).    The NPRO test may not be a suitable procedure to reveal such localized nitrosation in the stomach, and a more direct approach such as the determination of carcinogen-DNA adducts or DNA-damage in these lesions would be required.

New Approaches to Test the Hypothesis on NOC Formation and Gastric Carcinogenesis

Progress in laboratory methods development has produced a number of highly promising methods, some of which could be applied to test Correa's hypothesis. Table 3 presents examples of such methods that are currently available for monitoring humans and animals to carcinogens by analysis of carcinogen macromolecule adducts in tissues/fluids.

These methods have been applied to two different approaches to monitor macromolecule adducts.    One involves the quantitation of adducts in DNA or proteins of particular tissues (biopsy, autopsy material, placenta, blood cells) to provide useful information on the internal (biologically effective) dose of carcinogens. For example, Umbenhauer et al (47) and Wilt et al (51) applied a highly sensitive radioimmunoassay to detect $O^6$-methyldeoxyguanosine ($O^6$-medG) in DNA from human oesophageal and cardiac stomach mucosa from tissue samples obtained during surgery in Linxian County, People's Republic of China. Inhabitants of this area at high risk for both oesophageal and stomach cancer have been shown to be highly exposed to exogenous and endogenous NOC (22,23).    27 out of 37 tissue samples from Linxian County, showed high levels of $0^6$-medG (up to 160 fmol/mg DNA), whereas all 12 samples from hopsitals in Europe contained lower levels (below 45 fmol $0^6$-medG/mg DNA). The $^{32}$P-post labelling method, which detects carcinogen-modified DNA nucleotides that are post-labelled enzymatically with $^{32}$P, has also been applied to several human tissues such as buccal mucosa of betel nut chewers, placental tissues of smokers and non-smokers, colonic mucosa and blood lymphocytes (13,14,30,31,35). This method is extremely sensitive and can detect as little as one adduct per $10^9$ unmodified nucleotides in a small quantity of DNA. It could be potentially applicable to gastric biopsies, but the currently available method is limited to only bulky DNA adducts like aromatic hydrocarbons; this method does not provide structural information on unknown adducts.

Another promising approach is to quantitate excised DNA-adducts excreted in the urine. For example, aflatoxin $B_1$-DNA adducts have been determined in human urine by an immunoassay (15) and also by photon-counting synchronous fluorescence spectroscopy (1). Urinary excretion of alkylated DNA bases, eg 3-methyladenine (38) and 7-carboxymethylguanine (39) have been quantified in the urine of animals fed NOC such as nitrosodimethylamine and N-nitrosoglycocholic acid, a gastric carcinogen derived from nitrosated bile acid conjugate (5). Low levels of 3-methyladenine have been detected in human urine (40).

CONCLUSION

The methods listed in Table 3 can potentially be applicable to epidemiological field and clinical studies on gastric cancer. The NOC formation possibly occurring at the border of the normal and metaplastic areas of the stomach could only be demonstrated by analyzing modified DNA with those highly sensitive methods. Such studies are now in progress in this laboratory, in combination with assays for the determination of total NOC and the level of genotoxic agents in gastric juice using a new modified method (32) and bacterial genotoxicity tests, respectively (33). However, in order to further develop methods suitable for monitoring the exposure to gastric carcinogens, more studies are needed to identify the responsible carcinogens and thier macromolecule adducts. Several amino precursors, which show directly acting genotoxicity after in vitro nitrosation, have been identified in foods frequently consumed in high risk areas for stomach cancer. They include 4-chloro-6-methoxyindole in fava beans consumed in Colombia (52), some indole derivatives such as indole 3-acetonitrile in pickled chinese cabbage (48) and tyramine and beta-carboline derivativees in Japanese soya sauce (49). Also as recently found, smoked foods, whose frequent consumption has been associated with an increased risk of stomach cancer in Northern Europe (18), contain several compounds that are converted into directly-acting genotoxic substances after in vitro nitrosation (Ohshima et al, manuscript in preparation). Whether these precursors and other amide compounds are nitrosated by gastric bacteria should also be studied.

TABLE 3

SOME RECENTLY DEVELOPED ULTRA SENSITIVE TECHNIQUES FOR THE DETERMINATION OF DNA-ADDUCTS

| Methods | Type of Carcinogen/ DNA Lesion | Sensitivity (Adduct/Normal Nucleotides) | Comments |
|---|---|---|---|
| Radioimmunoassay ELISA | NOC, aflatoxins, PAH, oxidative damage | 1 in $10^7$-$10^8$ | Limited to known adducts |
| $^{32}$P-post labelling | PAH, aflatoxins (bulky adducts) | 1 in $10^7$-$10^{10}$ | Detection of known and unknown adducts |
| Synchronous excitation fluorescence spectroscopy | Aflatoxins, PAH | 1 in $10^5$ | Limited to fluorescent adducts |
| GC-MS (Negative ion chemical ionization) electron capturing derivatives | NOC, oxidative damage, etc | 1 in $10^8$ | Potentially capable of structure determination for unknown adducts |

Finally, there is a need to re-evaluate Correa's hypothesis of an increased formation of NOC under achlorhydria caused by CAG and IM, as a necessary condition for stomach cancer. Gastric carcinogens such as N-methyl-N-nitro-N'-nitrosoguanidine (MNNG) and its analogues (42) and nitrosated bile acid (5) have been shown to induce IM in the stomachs of experimental animals. This may suggest that NOC formed intragastrically by acid-catalyzed reaction in early life could play an important role in the initiation of gastric carcinogenesis, inducing gastric lesions such as IM In a later period of life. Moreover, since bacterial colonization has been shown to increase the incidence of gastric tumours induced by MNNG in experimental animals (4,26), bacteria may produce agents which act as co-carcinogens or tumour promoters. In relation, a specific type of bacteria, Campylobacter pylori, recently identified in human stomach mucosa as a possible aetiological agent of gastritis, may also contribute to gastric carcinogenesis by inducing chronic irritation or inflammation: the role of the chronic tissue injury has also been implicated in later stages of carcinogenesis, possibly through continuous generation of reactive oxygen species such as a superoxide anion and hydroxy radicals known to produce oxidative DNA base damage (4). Some methods (Table 3) may also be useful to detect such oxidative DNA damage, and future studies should take this end-point into consideration when investigating aetiological mechanisms leading to the intestinal type of gastric cancers.

## REFERENCES

1.  Autrup H, Bradley KA, Shamsuddin AKM, Wakhisi J, Wasunna A (1983) Carcinogenesis 4:1193-1195

2.  Bartsch H, Ohshima H, Munoz N, Crespi M, Lu SH (1983) In: Harris CC, Autrup HN (eds) Human Carcinogenesis. Academic Press, New York, pp833-855

3.  Bartsch H, Ohshima H, Munoz N, Crespi M, Ramazzotti V, Lambert R, Minaire Y, Forichon J, Walters CL (1984) In: O'Neill IK, von Borstel RC, Miller CT, Long J, Bartsch H (eds) N-nitroso compounds: occurrence, biological effects and relevance to human cancer (IARC Scientific Publications No 41). International Agency for Research on Cancer, Lyon pp955-962

4.  Blake DR, Allen RE, Lunic J (1987) Br Med Bull 43:371-385

5.  Busby WF, Shuker DEG, Charnley G, Newberne PM, Tannenbaum SR (1985) Cancer Res 45:1367-1371

6.  Calmels S, Ohshima H, Vincent P, Gounot AM, Bartsch H, (1985) Carcinogenesis 6:911-915

7.  Calmels S, Ohshima H, Bartsch (1988) J Gen Microbiol 134:221-226

8.  Charnley G, Tannenbaum SR, Correa P (1982) In: Magee PM (ed) Nitrosamines and human cancer Banbury Report 12. Cold Spring Harbor Laboratory Cold Spring Harbor NY, pp503-522

9.  Chen J, Ohshima H, Yang H, Li J, Campbell TC, Peto R, Bartsch H (1987) In: Bartsch H, O'Neill I, Schulte-Hermann R (eds) The relevance of N-nitroso compounds to human cancer, exposures and mechanisms (IARC Scientific Publications No 84). International Agency for Research on Cancer, Lyon pp503-506

10. Correa P, Haenszel W, Cuello C, Tannenbaum S, Archer M (1975) Lancet ii:58-60

11. Crespi M, Ohshima H, Ramazzotti V, Munoz N, Grassi A, Casale V, Leclerc H, Calmels S, Cattoen C, Kaldor J, Bartsch H (1987) In: Bartsch H, O'Neill I, Schulte-Hermann R (eds) The relevance of N-nitroso compounds to human cancer, exposures and mechanisms (IARC Scientific Publications No 84). International Agency for Research on Cancer, Lyon pp511-517

12. Druckrey H, Preussmann R, Ivankovic S, Schmahl D (1967) Z Krebsforsch 69:103-210

13. Dunn BP, Stich HF (1986) Carcinogenesis 7:1150-1120

14. Everson RB, Randerath E, Santella RM, Cefalo RC, Avitts TA, Randerath K (1986) Science 231:54-57

15. Groopmann JD (1988) In: Bartsch H, Hemminki K, O'Neill IK (eds) Methods for detecting DNA damaging agents in humans: application in cancer epidemiology and prevention (IARC Scientific Publications No 89). International Agency for Research on Cancer, Lyon (in press)

16. Hall CN, Kirkham JS, Northfield TC (1987) Gut 28:216-220

17. Hall CN, Darkin D, Viney N, Cook A, Kirkham JS, Northfield TC (1987) In: Bartsch H, O'Neill I, Schulte-Hermann R (eds) The relevance of N-nitroso compounds to human cancer, exposures and mechanisms (IARC Scientific Publications No 84). International Agency for Research on Cancer, Lyon, pp527-530

18. Howson CP, Hiyama T, Wynder EL (1986) Epidemiol Rev 8:1-27

19. Kamiyama S, Ohshima H, Shimada A, Saito N, Bourgade MC, Ziegler P, Bartsch H (1987) In: Bartsch H, O'Neill I, Schulte-Hermann R (eds) The relevance of N-nitroso compounds to human cancer, exposures and mechanisms (IARC Scientific Publications No 84). International Agency for Research on Cancer, Lyon pp497-502

20. Leach S, Cook A, Challis B, Hill MJ, Thompson M (1986) Cancer Lett 30 (Suppl) 527-528)

21. Leach SA, Thompson M, Hill M (1987) Carcinogenesis 8:1907-1912

22. Lu SH, Ohshima H, Fu H-M, Tian Y, Li F-M, Blettner M, Wahrendorf J, Bartsch H (1986) Cancer Res 46:1485-1491

23. Lu SH, Yang WX, Guo LP, Li FM, Wang GJ, Zhang JS, Li PZ (1987) In: Bartsch H, O'Neill I, Schulte-Hermann R (eds) The relevance of N-nitroso compounds to human cancer, exposures and mechanisms (IARC Scientific Publications No 84). International Agency for Research on Cancer, Lyon pp538-543

24. Mirvish SS (1983) J Natl Cancer Inst 71:629-647

25. Mirvish Ss, Sams J, Fan TY, Tannenbaum SR (1973) J Natl Cancer Inst 51:1833-1839

26. Morishita Y, Shimizu T (1983) Cancer Lett 77:347-352

27. Ohshima H, Bartsch H (1981) Cancer Res 41:3658-3662

28. Ohshima H, Mahon CAT, Wahrendorf J, Bartsch H (1983) Cancer Res 43:5072-5076

29. Parkin DM, Stjernsward J, Muir CS (1984) Bull WHO 62: 163-182

30. Phillips DH, Hewer A, Grover PL (1986) Carcinogenesis 7:2071-2075

31. Phillips DH, Hewer A, Grover PL, Jass JR (1988) In: Bartsch H, Hemminki K, O'Neill IK (eds) Methods for detecting DNA damaging agents in humans: application in cancer epidemiology and prevention (IARC Scientific Publication No 89). International Agency for Research on Cancer, Lyon (in press)

32. Pignatelli B, Richard I, Bourgade M-C, Bartsch H (1987) Analyst 112: 945-949

33. Pignatelli B, Calmels S, Malaveille C, Ohshima H, Munoz N, Bartsch H (1988) In the proceedings of "Campylobacter pylori" meeting, held in Nancy 16 January 1988 (in press)

34. Preussmann RAW, Tricker AR (1988) In: Reed PI, Hill MJ (eds) Gastric Carcinogenesis. Elsevier, Amsterdam pp

35. Randerath K, Miller RH, Mittal D, Randerath E (1988) In: Bartsch H, Hemminki, K, O'Neill IK (eds) Methods for detecting DNA damaging agents in humans: application in cancer epidemiology and prevention (IARC Scientific Publication No 89). International Agency for Research on Cancer, Lyon (in press)

36. Reed PI, Haines K, Smith PL, House FR, Walters CL (1981) Lancet ii:550-552

37. Schlag P, Ulrich H, Merkle P, Bockler R, Peter M, Herfarth C (1980) Lancet i:727-729

38. Shuker DEG, Bailey E, Farmer PB (1987) In: Bartsch H, O'Neill I, Schulte-Hermann R (eds) The relevance of N-nitroso compounds to human cancer, exposures and mechanisms (IARC Scientific Publication No 84). International Agency for Research on Cancer, Lyon, pp407-410

39. Shuker DEG, Howell JR, Street BW (1987) In: Bartsch H, O'Neill I, Schulte-Hermann R (eds) The relevance of N-nitroso compounds to human cancer, exposures and mechansims (IARC Scientific Publication No 84). Interntional Agency for Research on Cancer, Lyon pp187-190

40. Shuker DEG, Bailey T, Parry A, Lamb J, Farmer PB (1987) Carcinogenesis 8:956-962

41. Sugimura T, Fujimura S (1967) Nature 216:943-944

42. Sugimura T, Matsukura N, Sato S (1987) In: Bartsch H, Armstrong B (eds) Host factors in human carcinogenesis (IARC Scientific Publication No 39). International Agency for Research on Cancer, Lyon pp516-530

43. Sumi Y, Miyakawa M (1981) Gann 72:700-704

44. Tannenbaum SR, Archer MC, Wishnok JS, Correa P, Cuello C, Haenszel W (1977) In: Hiatt HH, Watson JD, Winsten JA (eds) Origins of human cancer Book C, Human risk assessment. Cold Spring Harbor Laboratory, Cold Spring Harbor NY, pp1609-1625

45. Tatsuta M, Okuda S, Tamura H, Taniguchi H, Tamura H (1979) Cancer 43:317-321

46. Toth B, Nagel D, Ross A (1982) Br J Cancer 46:417-422

47. Umbenhauer D, wild CP, Montesano R, Saffhill R, Boyle JM, Huh N, Kirstein U, Thomale J, Rajewsky MF, Lu SH (1985) Int J Cancer 36:661-665

48. Wakabayashi K, Nagao M, Ochiai M, Tahira T, Yamaizumi Z, Sugimura T (1985) Mut Res 143:17-21

49. Wakabayashi K, Nagao M, Ochiai M, Fujita Y, Tahira T, Nakayasu M, Ohgaki H, Takayama S, Sugimura T (1987) In: Bartsch H, O'Neill I, Schulte-Hermann R (eds) The relevance of N-nitroso compounds to human cancer, exposures and mechanisms (IARC Scientific Publication No 84). International Agency for Research on Cancer, Lyon pp287-291

50. Walters CL (1988) In: Reed PI, Hill MJ (eds) Gastric Carcinogenesis. Elsevier, Amsterdam pp

51. Wild CP, Umbenhauer D, Chapot B, Montesano R (1986) J Coll Biochem 30:171-179

52. Yang D, Tannenbaum SR, Buch G, Lee GCM (1984) Carcinogenesis 5:1219-1224

© Elsevier Science Publishers B.V. (Biomedical Division)
Gastric carcinogenesis. P.I. Reed, M.J. Hill, editors.

GASTRIC CARCINOGENESIS: LUMINAL FACTORS

MICHAEL J HILL

PHLS-CAMR, Porton Down, Salisbury, Wiltshire SP4 OJG, UK

INTRODUCTION

According to the model of gastric carcinogenesis proposed by Correa et al (10), the first stage is gastric atrophy which progresses to chronic atrophic gastritis. This results in decreased acid secretion to the point where the gastric luminal pH does not fall below 4 and therefore fails to sterilise the gastric contents; the consequence of this is that a resident bacterial flora becomes established in the stomach. It was hypothesised that this bacterial flora reduced dietary nitrate to nitrite and catalysed the formation of N-nitroso compounds; these latter carcinogens were hypothesised to be responsible for the progression through intestinal metaplasia, then increasingly severe dysplasia to gastric carcinoma of the intestinal type. If this hypothesis is correct then the gastric juice luminal factors should be important risk factors for gastric carcinogenesis.

The luminal factors of interest are the gastric bacterial flora, the major precursors of N-nitroso compound formation (nitrite and nitrosatable nitrogen compounds), the N-nitroso compounds themselves, and also the components of bile (particularly the bile acids) that have also been implicated in gastric carcinogenesis. Bile reflux has been discussed in detail in this symposium by Mortensen (28) whilst the N-nitroso compounds have been covered in the papers by Preussmann (31) and Walters (43). This paper will be limited to consideration of the bacterial flora, nitrate, nitrite and nitrosatable nitrogen compounds. These will be discussed in turn, then the evidence that they are important risk factors in gastric carcinogenesis will be reviewed.

THE LUMINAL FACTORS

The Gastric Bacterial Flora

Most of the normal commensal flora of man and other animals cannot metabolise at pH values below 4 and are consequently killed by such acidic conditions. Since the normal stomach has a pH of 2 the normal gastric lumen is either sterile or contains organisms that are barely able to survive. In contrast the achlorhydric stomach has been known for decades to be populated by a complex bacterial flora (46) rich in both salivary and faecal-type organisms. As bacteriological techniques have improved, particularly the methods for the isolatin and enumeration of the strictly anaerobic oxygen-sensitive genera, the apparent complexity of the flora of the achlorhydric stomach has increased; Table 1 lists the major species reported by Drasar et al (12), by Forsythe et al (13) and other sources.

TABLE 1

THE BACTERIAL FLORA OF THE ACHLORHYDRIC STOMACH, WITH ITS ABILITY TO REDUCE NITRATE AND NITRITE (DATA FROM VARIOUS SOURCES)

| Bacterial Group | Numbers Present | Relative Enzymic Activites | |
|---|---|---|---|
| | | Nitrate reductase | Nitrite reductase |
| Strep. salivarius | $10^6$-$10^8$ | - | - |
| Other oral streptococci | ++ | - | $\pm$ |
| Faecal streptococci | $10^4$ | ++ | + |
| Staphylococci and micrococci | $10^4$-$10^6$ | ++ | ++ |
| Veillonella spp. | $10^4$-$10^6$ | +++ | + |
| Neisseria spp. | ++ | $\pm$ | +++ |
| Lactobacillus spp. | $10^4$-$10^6$ | ++ | ++ |
| Bacteroides fragilis | $\pm$ | - | - |
| B. asaccharolyticus | $10^2$-$10^6$ | - | - |
| Enterobacteria | ++ | +++ | ++ |
| Pseudomonas spp. | + | ++ | ++ |
| Haemophilus spp. | $\pm$ | ++ | + |
| Corynebacterium spp. | $\pm$ | ++ | ++ |
| Fusobacterium spp. | + | ++ | ++ |

In the context of the hypothesis of Correa et al (10), the important chracteristics of this flora are (a) its ability to reduce nitrate to nitrite, and (b) its ability to catalyse the N-nitrosation reaction.

Nitrate reductase activity. A wide range of bacterial species can reduce nitrate to nitrite, including many of those reported int he gastric bacterial flora (Table 1). Nitrate reductase allows nitrate to be used as an alternative electron acceptor to atmospheric oxygen and so requires anaerobic conditions both for its production and its activity. The enzyme from Esch. coli has an activity related to the amount of cytochrome b1. Nitrate is degraded by two major pathways, namely nitrate assimilation and nitrate dissimulation (or nitrate respiration). In the former, nitrate is reduced to nitrite then through ammonia which can then be incorporated into bacterial protein. In the latter pathway the main function of nitrate reductase is to act as an electron acceptor and an energy source.

A proportion of organisms produce a nitrite reductase which, if present at high activity in the stomach, would decrease the nitrite concentration. Forsythe et al (13), in a study of patients with pernicious anaemia and hypogammaglobulinaemia (HGG), were able to relate the nitrite concentration in gastric juice to the proportion of strains producing nitrate reductase relative to those producing nitrite reductase.

N-nitrosation by bacteria. The ability of bacteria, particularly Esch. coli, to catalyse the N-nitrosation reaction was first reported by Sander (35) and confirmed subsequently by Hawksworth and Hill (15) and by many other groups. Until recently there has been considerable disagreement concerning the mechanism of this catalysis; some claimed that the catalysis was enzymic whilst others have been of the opinion that the bacteria merely generated the nitrite and the acid conditions required for the acid-catalysed nitrosation. As is usual in such disputes, it is likely that both are correct. Undoubtedly many species of nitrate-reducing bacteria also ferment sugars to yield pH values of, for example, below 5.5; at such pH values the acid-catalysed reaction still proceeds although at well below the optimum rates achieved at pH 2. However, Leach et al (23) and Calmels et al (3) have demonstrated beyond dispute that bacteria are able to produce an enzyme capable of catalysing N-nitrosation. Further, Leach et al (24) have shown that, whereas the coliform organisms and other nitrate assimilators have a relatively low "N-nitrosatase", the activity in some nitrate dissimilating strains (e.g. Pseudomonas spp., Neisseria spp.) is higher by orders of magnitude (Table 2). Calmels et al (4) have shown that, in Esch. coli the enzyme appears to be related to nitrate reductase. Thus, the presence of a gastric bacterial flora per se is relatively less important than its nitrate reductase activity and the presence of nitrate dissimilating species (25).

## Gastric Juice Nitrate and Nitrite

Hawksworth et al (16) showed that the concentration of nitrite in the gastric juice was very much higher in patients with achlorhydria than in control persons with a normal acid stomach; this has been confirmed subsequently by Ruddell et al (33) and numerous other groups. Table 3 lists typical concentrations of gastric juice nitrate and nitrite in various groups of patients. It is essential to measure both nitrate and nitrite; a low nitrite concentration may be due to either (a) a low activity of nitrate reductase, or (b) a low concentration of nitrate precursor, or (c) a high activity of nitrite reductase, and it may be important to be able to distinguish between these alternatives. In general, the availability of nitrate in the stomach is not the factor limiting the nitrite concentration, and in patients where the pH is high and the concentration of both nitrate and of nitrite is low the usual explanation

TABLE 2

RATE OF N-NITROSATION BY VARIOUS BACTERIAL SPECIES (DATA FROM LEACH ET AL (23), VARIOUS SOURCES)

| Non-denitrifying Species | Rate* | Denitrifying Species | Rate |
|---|---|---|---|
| Esch. coli strain: | | Ps. aeruginosa strain: | |
| BM1056 | 28 | BM1030 | 12000 |
| BM1023 | 58 | BM1035 | 5000 |
| BM1042 | 20 | BM1233 | 660 |
| BM1033 | 0 | | |
| BM1047 | 0 | Neisseria spp. strain: | |
| BM1046 | 0 | 2-10 | 1300 |
| | | 3-10 | 240 |
| | | 1-10 | 660 |
| Streptococcus spp. strain | 0 | 2-20 | 260 |
| BM6 | | | |
| Veillonella spp. strain: | | | |
| 2V | 0 | Alc. faecalis NCTC415 | 2300 |
| 24 | 0 | | |
| | | B. licheniformis NCTC8721 | 1620 |
| Clostridium spp. strain: | | | |
| 8 | 0 | | |
| F | 0 | | |
| Bifidobacterium spp. | 0 | | |
| strain 10 | | | |

*Rate is in nmol N-nitrosomorpholine produced/mg protein/hour is the high activity of both nitrate reductase and nitrite reductase in the gastric bacterial flora.

TABLE 3

GASTRIC JUICE NITRATE AND NITRITE IN VARIOUS PATIENT GROUPS
(DATA ACCUMULATED FROM VARIOUS SOURCES)

| Patient Group | Concentration in Gastric Juice | | |
|---|---|---|---|
| | Nitrate (uMol/l) | Nitrite (uMol/l) | N-nitroso Compounds (nM/l) |
| Duodenal ulcer (DU) | 339 $\pm$ 51 | 1.5 $\pm$ 0.7 | 159 $\pm$ 48 |
| Gastric ulcer | 268 $\pm$ 56 | 5.9 $\pm$ 4.7 | 109 $\pm$ 54 |
| DU on cimetidine | 278 $\pm$ 74 | 52.0 $\pm$ 20.8 | 237 $\pm$ 41 |
| Hypogammaglobinaemia | 144 | 135 | ND |
| Pernicious anaemia - Study A | 209 $\pm$ 42 | 59 $\pm$ 13 | ND |
| - Study B | 35 | 47 | ND |
| - Study C | ND | 120 $\pm$ 20 | ND |
| Partial gastrectomy 187 $\pm$ 180 | 52 $\pm$ 70 | ND | |

Nitrosatable Nitrogen Compounds

The availability of nitrosatable nitrogen compounds is rarely likely to be the limiting factor determining the rate of formation of N-nitroso compounds in the stomach. Shepherd et al (38) and Kawabata et al (20) demonstrated that the diet contains a rich variety of nitrosatable nitrogen compounds, although Kawabata et al (20) reported that they were unable to find large amounts of any single compound. It is likely, therefore, that the substrates of endogenous origin are present in gastric juice in very much greater amounts than those from the diet. In order to obtain an estimate of the amount of nitrosatable nitrogen compound in gastric juice, Walters et al (44) carried out an exhaustive nitrosation of pooled gastric juice and demonstrated that, using Walters' assay for total N-nitroso compounds, the amount of nitrosatable nitrogen compound was 10-20ug/ml. Since in the achlorhydric stomach the concentration of total N-nitroso compound was in the range 0.1-2uMol/l, the proportion of available nitrosatable nitrogen actually N-nitrosated in the achlorhydric stomach was normally about 1 to 10%.

LUMINAL FACTORS AND GASTRIC CARCINOGENESIS

If the Correa model of gastric carcinogenesis is correct then (a) gastric achlorhydria in any situation is associated with an increased risk of gastric cancer,

(b) an increased gastric pH should be associated with an increased concentration in the gastric juice of bacteria (particularly nitrate reducing bacteria), nitrite and N-nitroso compounds, and (c) the gastric juice analyses should be related to the gastric histopathology, particularly the severity of epithelial dysplasia. Further, if gastric carcinogenesis is caused by N-nitroso compounds formed locally in the gastric lumen then, since N-nitroso compounds are either locally acting or target-organ specific, and since it is unlikely that only the locally acting compounds would be formed, cancers at other sites should also be common in persons with disease states associated with hypochlorhydria. Finally, there should be an increased risk of intestinal-type cancer of the stomach in populations with a high intake of dietary nitrate. These will be considered in turn.

## Gastric Achlorhydria and Gastric Cancer

Precancerous and precursor lesions in gastric carcinogenesis have been discussed in detail elsewhere in this symposium by Correa (9). For the purpose of this chapter, it is sufficient that all of the diseases known to be associated with gastric hypoacidity (e.g. gastric atrophy, chronic atrophic gastritis, intestinal metaplasia, Polya partial gastrectomy, Billroth I partial gastrectomy, vagotomy of varying degrees of selectivity, pernicious anaemia, hypogammaglobulinaemia) carry an excess risk of gastric cancer ranging from 2-4 (gastric atrophy) to more than 50-fold (HGG) as shown in Table 4. This is in agreement with the hypothesis of Correa.

## Gastric Juice Analyses and pH

It has been known for more than 60 years that the achlorhydric stomach is heavily colonised with a rich bacterial flora (46) and these results have been confirmed and extended since the development of techniques for the quantitative recovery of the oxygen-sensitive component of the flora. Hawksworth et al (16) carried out a study of gastric juice analyses in the context of the possible role of N-nitroso compounds in gastric cancer; they demonstrated that an elevated gastric pH was accompanied by an increased gastric bacterial flora, particularly the nitrate-reducing bacteria, and by an increased nitrite concentration. Ruddell et al confirmed and extended these results and showed that the gastric juice analyses were elevated in the hypochlorhydric stomach in general (33) and more specifically in patients with pernicious anaemia (34). The results were presented and discussed in the context of gastric carcinogenesis. Since then more than 20 studies (Table 5) have demonstrated that in the hypochlorhydric stomach there is a profuse bacterial flora and an increased nitrite concentration regardless of the cause of the hypoacidity. This is in support of the hypothesis of Correa et al (10).

TABLE 4

THE RELATIVE RISK OF GASTRIC CANCER IN PERSONS WITH DISEASE STATES CHARACTERISED BY LOSS OF GASTRIC ACIDITY (FOR DETAILS AND REFERENCES SEE (18))

| Disease State | Risk of Gastric Cancer in Relation to that in the Normal Population |
|---|---|
| Gastric atrophy | Increased risk |
| Chronic atrophic gastritis | Risk increased 2-3 fold |
| Intestinal metaplasia | Risk increased 2-4 fold |
| Pernicious anaemia | Risk increased 3-6 fold |
| Hypogammaglobinaemia | Risk increased 50 fold |
| Gastric surgery* | |
| Billroth 1 gastrectomy | Risk increased 3-6 fold |
| Polya gastrectomy | Risk increased 3-6 fold |
| Vagotomy and drainage | Risk increased 10 fold |
| Selective vagotomy | Risk increased? |

*After 20 years latency

Gastric Juice Analyses and Gastric Histopathology

In a number of reports the gastric juice analyses have been related to the gastric histopathology, particularly the severity of epithelial dysplasia (Table 6). These have shown a correlation between the severity of epithelial dysplasia and both the bacterial flora and the concentration of nitrite in the gastric juice; until the analytical problems have been resolved the very important question of the relation between gastric epithelial dysplasia and the concentration of N-nitroso compounds cannot be answered. Nevertheless, the results summarised in Table 6 support the Correa hypothesis.

Gastric Achlorhydria and Other Cancers

If the relationships in Table 1 are caused by the local production of locally acting N-nitroso compounds, it is possible that other classes of organotropic N-nitroso compounds might also be formed. If this is so then gastric achlorhydria should be associated with cancers at sites other than the stomach. This has been studied in gastric surgery patients and in patients with pernicious anaemia.

TABLE 5

THE RELATION BETWEEN GASTRIC JUICE pH AND GASTRIC JUICE ANALYSES
IN VARIOUS STUDIES

| Reference No | Patient Groups | Effect of Increased pH Bacterial Flora | Nitrite Conc. |
|---|---|---|---|
| 12 | Various | Increased | |
| 33 | Various | Increased | Increased |
| 34 | PA and Controls | Increased | Increased |
| 19 | PG | | Increased |
| 44 | Various | Increased | Increased |
| 36 | PG | Increased | Increased |
| 1 | PA and Controls | Increased | Increased |
| 37 | PG | Increased | Increased |
| 32 | Various | Increased | Increased |
| 30 | Various | Increased | Increased |
| 26 | Persons on Cimetidine | Increased | Increased |
| 45 | Various | Increased | Increased |
| 21 | Surgery for DU | Increased | Increased |
| 39 | PA and Control | Increased | Increased |
| 11 | PA Immune Deficient and Controls | Increased | Increased |
| 6 | PG and Controls | Increased | Increased |
| 14 | PG, PA, Control | Increased | Increased |
| 29 | PG | Increased | Increased |
| 47 | Normal Persons with Various Gastric pH | Increased | Increased |
| 40 | Various | Increased | Increased |
| 8 | Cimetidine or Ranitidine or Control | Increased | Increased |
| 22 | Various | Increased | Increased |
| 5 | Surgery for Ulcer | Increased | Increased |
| 41 | Ranitidine or Control | Increased | Increased |

Caygill et al (6) studied a group of 348 peptic ulcer patients treated by Polya partial gastrectomy. There was no excess risk of cancer at any site during the first 20 years post-operation but, subsequently, there was an excess risk of cancer of the stomach, biliary tract and colorectum. In a much larger study of 5018 patients treated surgically for peptic ulcer (7) there was the same latent period of 20 years with no excess risk of cancer at any site, followed in subsequent years by an excess risk of cancer of the stomach, biliary tract, colorectum, and some other sites (Table 7). In a study of approximately 1000 patient with pernicious anaemia by Caygill et al (6) the results were similar to those obtained with the gastric surgery cases; in addition to the excess risk of gastric cancer observed by others there was also an excess risk of cancer of the biliary tract and of the large bowel. Again this is consistent with the hypothesis that N-nitroso compounds formed in the gastric lumen are responsible, at least in part, for the progression from gastric atrophy to gastric cancer.

TABLE 6

THE RELATION BETWEEN GASTRIC JUICE ANALYSES AND GASTRIC HISTOPATHOLOGY IN PATIENTS WITH HYPOACIDITY OF VARIOUS ETIOLOGIES

| References | Patient Group | Observation |
|---|---|---|
| Jones et al (19) | Gastric surgery patients | Nitrite concentration correlated with the severity of dysplasia |
| Watt et al (45) | Various | Bacterial flora and nitrite concentration correlated with the severity of dysplasia |
| Mortensen et al (29) | Gastric surgery patients | Nitrite concentration correlated with the severity of dysplasia |
| Hall et al (14) | pernicious anaemia gastric surgery and controls | nitrite concentration correlated with the severity of epithelial dysplasia |

196

TABLE 7

RISK OF CANCER AT VARIOUS SITES FOLLOWING GASTRIC SURGERY FOR PEPTIC ULCER AND RELATED TO THE TIME INTERVAL POST-SURGERY (DATA FROM CAYGILL ET AL, 1987)

| Site of Cancer | Relative Risk in Relation to the Number of Years Post-Surgery | |
|---|---|---|
| | 0-20 Years | More than 20 Years |
| Stomach | 1.2 | 4.5 |
| Colorectum | 0.7 | 1.6 |
| Biliary Tract | 1.9 | 8.6 |
| Oesophagus | 0.8 | 2.3 |
| Bladder | 0.6 | 2.4 |
| Pancreas | 0.7 | 3.8 |
| Breast | 0.5 | 4.0 |

Nitrate Intake and Gastric Cancer

There have been many reports of a relation between nitrate intake and gastric cancer incidence (Table 8); the correlations have been strongest where the gastric cancer risk is highest and where, therefore, the proportion of intestinal-type cancers is likely to be highest. Mirvish (27) showed that, in a study of 12 populations, the gastric cancer incidence was correlated with the nitrate intake.

In many of the studies in Table 8 the source of the high nitrate intake has been the drinking water. There is considerable confusion in the literature caused by the misuse of data of public health importance in the gastric carcinogenesis debate. In public health studies it is necessary to examine the health risk associated with the analysis of water as currently consumed. In studies of gastric carcinogenesis it is necessary to contrast the risk of the disease in populations consuming greatly different amounts of nitrate. Under normal conditions drinking water contributes only 0-15% of the total nitrate intake and so variations in such low levels do not affect significantly the total nitate intake. The numerous studies showing no relation between gastric cancer incidence and variations in such low nitrate concentrations in drinking water (eg 2,42), although providing valuable reassurance to the general public, give no information on the role of nitrate in gastric carcinogenesis and are, indeed, irrelevent to that discussion. When the nitrate concentration exceeds the WHO recommended limit of 50mg/l, drinking water becomes the major contributor to the total nitrate intake and significantly increases it; in all of the studies cited in Table 8 relating high nitrate in drinking water to gastric cancer risk, the nitrate concentration was close to or above 100mg/l.

TABLE 8

THE RELATION BETWEEN HIGH NITRATE INTAKE AND GASTRIC CANCER RISK (FOR DETAILS AND REFERENCES SEE HILL, 1984)

| Country | Prevalance of Gastric Atrophy | Source of the High Nitrate Exposure |
|---------|-------------------------------|-------------------------------------|
| Chile | High | Vegetables, due to high use of nitrate fertiliser |
| Colombia | High | Vegetables and water, due to the high nitrate content of the soil |
| China | High | Vegetables, due to the low molybdenum content of the soil |
| Japan | High | Vegetables, due to the high nitrate content of the soil |
| Hungary | Intermediate | Drinking water (much greater than 100mg/l) |
| Italy | Intermediate | Drinking water |
| Israel | Low | Drinking water (greater than 100mg/l) |
| England | Low | Drinking water, (almost 100mg/l) |
| Denmark | Low | Drinking water |

CONCLUSIONS

Since the stomach is the first resting place of all food and drinks, it is inevitable that it will be exposed to a wide range of carcinogens and that, therefore, gastric cancer will have a multifactorial aetiology. Nevertheless, there is now a large body of evidence relating gastric luminal factors, particularly the gastric bacterial flora and the nitrite concentration, to the progression from atrophic gastritis through intestinal metaplasia, increasingly severe dysplasia to gastric cancer.

ACKNOWLEDGEMENTS

The work of this laboratory is financially supported by the Cancer Research Campaign.

REFERENCES

1.  Bartholomew B, Hill MJ, Hudson MJ et al (1980) IARC Scientific Publication number 31: p595-608
2.  Beresford SA (1985) Int J Epidemiol 34: 57-63

198

3. Calmels S, Ohshima H, Vincent P et al (1985) Carcinogenesis 6: 911-915

4. Calmels S, Ohshima H, Rosenkranz E et al (1987) Carcinogenesis 8: 1085-1087

5. Carboni M, Guadagni S, Pistoia M et al (1986) Scand J Gastro 21: 461-470

6. Caygill CPJ, Craven J, Hall R et al (1984) IARC Scientific Publication Number 57: 895-900

7. Caygill CPJ, Hill MJ, Hall CN et al (1987) Gut 28: 924-8

8. Cook AR, Hill MJ, Hall N et al (1985) Brit J Cancer 52: 446

9. Correa P (1988) In: Reed PI, Hill MJ (eds) Gastric Carcinogenesis, elsevier, Amsterdam pp

10. Correa P, Haensel W, Cuello C, Tannenbaum S, Archer M (1975) Lancet ii: 58-60

11. Dolby J, Webster A, Borriello SP et al (1984) Scand J Gastroenterol 19: 105-110

12. Drasar BS, Shiner M, McLeod GM (1969) Gastroenterology 56: 71-77

13. Forsythe S, Cole JA (1987) J Gen Microbiol 133: 1845-1849

14. Hall CN, Cook AR, Darkin D et al (1984) Clin Science 66: 34P-35P

15. Hawksworth GM, Hill MJ (1971) Brit J Cancer 25: 520-526

16. Hawksworth GM, Hill MJ, Gordillo G, Cuello C (1975) IARC Scientific Publication Number 9: p229-234

17. Hill MJ (1984) Clinics In Oncology 2: 237-249

18. Hill MJ (1986) Microbes and Human Carcinogenesis. Edward Arnold, London

19. Jones SM, Davies PW, Savage A (1978) Lancet 1: 1355

20. Kawabata T, Ohshima H, Uibu J, Nakamura M, Matsui M, Hamano M (1979) In "Naturally Occurring Carcinogens - Mutagens and Modulators of Carcinogenesis" (ed EC Miller et al) Jap Sci Soc Press, Tokyo, p195-209

21. Keighley M, Youngs D, Poxon V et al (1984) Gut 25: 238-245

22. Kyrtopoulos SA, Daskalakis G, Legakis NI and 7 other (1985) Carcinogenesis 6: 1135-1140

23. Leach S, Challis B, Cook AR, Hill MJ, Thompson MH (1985) Trans Biochem Soc 13: 380-381

24. Leach S, Cook A, Challis A, Hill M, Thompson M (1986) Cancer Lett 30: 527-528

25. Leach S, Thompson M, Hill M (1987) Carcinogenesis 8: 1907-1912

26. Milton-Thompson G, Lightfood N, Ahmet Z et al (1982) Lancet i: 1091-1094

27. Mirvish SS (1987) Cancer 58: 1842-1850

28. Mortensen N (1988) In: Reed PI, Hill MJ (eds) Gastric Carcinogenesis, Elsevier, Amsterdam pp

29. Mortensen N, Thomas WE, Cooper MJ et al (1984) Brit J Surg 71: 363

30. Muscroft TJ, Deane SA, Young D, Burdon DW, Keighley MRB (1981) Br J surg 68: 560-564

31. Preussmann R, Tricker AR (1988) In: Reed PI, Hill MJ (eds) Gastric Carcinogenesis, Elsevier, Amsterdam pp

32. Reed PI, Smith PL, Haines K et al 91981) Lancet ii: 550-552

33. Ruddell WSJ, Bone ES, Hill MJ, Blendis LM, Walters CL (1976) Lancet ii: 1037-1039

34. Ruddell WSJ, Bone ES, Hill MJ, Walters CL (1978) Lancet i: 521-523

35. Sander J (1968) Z Physiol Chem 439: 429-432

36. Schlag P, Bockler R, ulrich H et al (1980) Lancet i: 727-729

37. Schumpelick V, Schassan HH (1980) Langenbecks Arch Chir 350: 271-279

38. Shepherd SE, Schlatter C, Lutz WK (1987) Food Chem Toxicol 25: 91-108

39. Stockbrugger R, Cotton P, Menon G et al (1984) Scand J Gastro 19: 355-364

40. Stockbrugger R (1985) Scand J Gastroenterol 20 (Supplement 111): 7-15

41. Thomas JM, Misiewicz JJ, Cook AR et al (1987) Gut 28: 726-738

42. Vincent P, Dubois G, Leclerq H (1983) Rev Epidemiol Sante Publique 31: 199-207

43. Walters CL (1988) In: Reed PI, Hill MJ (eds) Gastric Carcinogenesis, Elsevier, Amsterdam pp

44. Walters CL, Hill MJ, Ruddell WSJ (1978) IARC Scientific Publication Number 19: 279-288

45. Watt PC, Patterson CC, Kennedy TL (1984) Brit Med J 288: 1335-1338

46. Wichels P (1924) Z Clin Med 100: 535-542

47. Zhang RF, Sun HL, Jin M-L, Li S-N (1984) Chinese Med J 97: 322-332

© Elsevier Science Publishers B.V. (Biomedical Division)
Gastric carcinogenesis. P.I. Reed, M.J. Hill, editors.

BILE AND ENTEROGASTRIC REFLUX - A FACTOR IN GASTRIC CANCER?

NEIL MORTENSEN[1] and PAUL HOUGHTON[2]
John Radcliffe Hospital, Oxford[1] and Bristol Royal Infirmary[2], UK

William Beaumont's observations on his famous patient with a fistula Alexis St Martin, demonstrated human duodenogastric reflux for the first time in 1833 (2). Later in the 1880s after the early gastroenterostomy operations bile vomiting was recognised as a serious and potentially lethal complication (14), and techniques were quickly developed to prevent bile reflux including the Roux-en-Y operation described by Cesar Roux in 1897 (35). The damaging effect of bile on gastric mucosa was first confirmed experimentally by Smith (40) who produced gastric ulcers by injecting bile and 0.5% hydrochloric acid into the stomach of dogs and cats. Since then the potential role of duodenogastric or bile reflux has been a popular hypothesis in the development of both benign and malignant gastric mucosal disease, particularly in the post-operative stomach.

The major problem in assessing the part played by reflux is that it is intermittent and unpredictable. Furthermore bile and duodenogastric reflux are not synonymous, and activated pancreatic enzymes or their added effect together with bile salts may be just as important. The retrograde passage of duodenal contents into the stomach is a normal physiological occurrence, both during fasting and after a meal, but the refluxate is usually rapidly cleared (19). These events have been demonstrated by both direct sampling techniques and non-invasive methods with isotopes (19,30,43). Labelling bile with an isotope has added a further complication to the reflux equation and, surprisingly, patients with non functioning gall bladders have greater degrees of reflux than those with a normal gall bladder (12). If the duodenal contents are to damage gastric mucosa then there would have to be either greater than normal reflux, impaired gastric emptying and clearance, an increased toxicity of the refluxate, or decreased gastric mucosal defences. Many studies have concentrated on the quantity of reflux.

EXPERIMENTAL STUDIES

Most experimental studies have used a carcinogen in combination with an operative technique to study the promoting effect of reflux. Morganstern (27) implanted 20-methyl-cholanthrene impregnated cotton threads into the gastric wall of rats with a gastroenterostomy either alone or combined with a vagotomy, and found an increased tumour yield. The incidence of experimental cancer using N-methyl-N[1]-butri-N-nitrosoguanidine is lower in animals without reflux (7,18) or treated by Roux-en-Y diversion (18,37). Tumour yield also increases when bile salts are given orally or bile is diverted into the stomach (21). Even in animals not treated with a carcinogen, duodenogastric reflux causes gastric carcinoma within 9 months in some studies (23) and this would be equivalent to the 20 years onset of gastric stump cancer in humans. Mason has found that pancreaticoduodenal secretions rather than bile are responsible for the increase but this is controversial (26). Attempts to study the effects of reflux on premalignant changes in experimental animals have been hampered by differences in the sequence of neoplastic transformation compared to human gastric mucosa. Mucosal proliferation as measured by DNA content and crypt cell production rate is increased as a result of reflux in both animals (18) and man (1) and by analogy with the colon and pancreas increased cell proliferation could promote gastric carcinogenesis.

## Clinical Studies

In the intact stomach bile concentrations in gastric aspirates are higher in patients with gastric ulcer than in controls, but there is considerable overlap with the normal range (3,15). In gastric cancer patients tumours in the antrum will affect both reflux and emptying and there are no good data on intragastric bile concentrations here. After surgery reflux may occur more readily, and the post operative stomach has been a particularly fruitful model for studying the effects of various factors on gastric mucosal changes. Domelloff (10) found bile reflux samples in Billroth II gastrectomy patients had 10 to 20% of the concentrations found in human hepatic bile. Since there is an association between gastric surgery for peptic ulcer and the subsequent development of stump cancer 20 or more years later reflux has been implicated in the development of human gastric cancer (10,28,36,39,41). Coupled with gastric carcinogenesis are a series of premalignant histological changes including atrophic gastritis, intestinal metaplasia and dysplasia. Whilst the relationship between these changes and the development of cancer is not clear, these are more common in post-gastrectomy patients (28,36,39). Du Plessis first suggested that reflux caused the chronic gastritis commonly seen after partial gastrectomy, and in a group of 50 patients with severe reflux Domelloff (10) found 4 with either cancer or severe dysplasia. There is a correlation between the quantity of bile reflux and the degree of gastritis (41) and other mucosal changes assessed by single samples (35) but these have been criticised as being unrepresentative (3) and there are variations depending on whether or not the subject is recumbent or has eaten a meal. Houghton (17) found total bile acid levels in gastric aspirates to be higher in patients with atrophic gastritis, intestinal metaplasia and dysplasia, but not chronic gastritis.

The severity of dysplasia, however, did not correlate with total bile acid levels. Free bile acid levels were higher in those with atrophic gastritis. Gastric dysplasia improves after bile diversion, although gastritis, gastric atrophy and intestinal metaplasia do not, suggesting that these changes may be irreversible (16,29,39,45). Foveolar hyperplasia is increased with bile reflux and also improved following Roux-en-Y diversion (35). All these changes are less common after other forms of peptic ulcer surgery.

## MECHANISMS OF REFLUX IN GASTRIC CARCINOGENESIS

Exposure of the gastric mucosa to duodenal contents produces erosions and ulcers, and these can be prevented by a long Roux-en-Y (20,24). Pure pancreatic juice is less damaging than pure bile (29) and some have suggested that alkaline duodenal juice may moderate the severity of gastritis (9,31). In animal studies bile salts even in low concentrations have been shown to alter the properties of gastric mucus and to inhibit alkali secretion by gastric mucosa (34). This would allow back diffusion of acid, and the surface epithelial layer could then be damaged by topical bile acids (4). Their detergent action on the mucus barrier may allow luminal carcinogens to act on exposed stem cells once epithelial cells have been shed (10). Lysolecithin is formed spontaneously from the hydrolysis of biliary lecithin by pancreatic phospholipase and is highly cytotoxic (31) and might have a co-promotional role with bile. It too is found in greater concentrations in post-gastrectomy patients than in those after other forms of gastric surgery (8). Bile acids can induce sarcomas but not carcinomas when injected into experimental animals (5,22).

Drasar and Hill (11) have suggested that nitrate reducing bacteria in the achlorhydric stomach might react with refluxing bile acids to form the carcinogen dimethylnitrosamine. N-nitroso bile acid conjugates are as mutagenic as MNNG but there is no evidence that they are actually carcinogens (32). Human gut flora can change bile acids and neutral sterols to a form resembling carcinogenic polycyclic aromatic hydrocarbons (6). Bacterial conjugation increases the concentration of membrane active free bile acids like the colonic promoter deoxycholic acid and the promoter and comutagen lithocholic acid (33).

In Domellof's group of 50 partial gastrectomy patients 85% had intragastric bacteria - usually coliforms (10). Clostridia have also been found in the post operative stomach, (43) and these are known to cause dehydrogenation and dehydroxylation of bile acids (25).

So bile salts or other constituents of duodenal juice could play a role in gastric carcinogenesis, as one factor in a series of factors, particularly after partial gastrectomy where the link seems the most plausible.

REFERENCES

1.  Assad RT, Eastwood GL (1980) Gastroenterology 79: 801-811

2.  Beaumont W (1833) Experiments and observation on the gastric juice, and the physiology of digestion. Plattsburgh , F P Allen

3.  Black RB, Roberts G, Rhodes J (1971) Gut 12: 552-558

4.  Carter KJ, Farley PC, Ritchie WP (1984) Surgery 96: 196-201

5.  Cook JW, Kennaway EL, Kennaway NM (1940) Nature 145: 627

6.  Coombs MM, Bhatt TS, Croft CJ (1973) Cancer Res 33: 832-837

7.  Dahm K, Eichen R, Mitschke H (1977) Langenbecks Arch Chir 344: 71-82

8.  Dewar P, King R, Johnson D (1982) Gut 23: 569-577

9.  Diserens H, Kestic R, Burri B, Mosimann F, Mosimann R (1984) Scand J Gastroenterol 19: 133-135

10.  Domellof L, Reddy BS, Weisburger JH (1980) Am J Surg 140: 291-295

11.  Drasar BS, Hill MJ (1974) Ac Press London: 193-225

12.  Drumm J, Donovan IA, Haider Z, Harding LK (1985) Br J Surg 72: 411

13.  Du Plessis DJ (1962) S Afr Med J 36: 471-478

14.  Earlam R (1983) Br J Surg 70: 393-397

15.  Frizis HI, Whitfield PF, Hobsley M (1985) Br J Surg 72: 411

16.  Hoare AM, McLeish A, Thompson H, Alexander-Williams J (1978) Gut 19: 163-165

17.  Houghton PWJ, Mortensen NJMcC, Thomas WEG, Cooper MJ, Morgan AP, Burton P (1986) Br J Surg 73: 354-356

18.  Houghton PWJ, Mortensen NJMcC, Williamson RCN (1987) Br J Surg 74: 288-291

19.  Keane FB, Dimagno EP, Malagelada JR (1981) Gastroenterology 81: 726-731

20.  Kirk RM (1970) Br J Surg 57: 521-524

21.  Kobori O, Shimizu T, Maeda M et al (1984) J Nat Canc Inst 73: 853-861

22.  Laccassagne A, Buu-Hoi NP, Zajdela F (1966) Nature 209: 1026-1027

23.  Langhans P, Heger RA, Hohenstein J, Bunte H (1987) Hepato Gastroenterol 28: 34-37

24.  Lawson HH (1964) Lancet 1: 469-472

25.  Lewis R, Gorbach S (1972) Arch Intern Med 130: 545-549

26.  Mason RC (1986) Br J Surg 73: 801-803

27.  Morgenstern L (1968) Arch Surg 96: 920-923

28.  Mortensen NJMcC, Thoms WEG, Jones SM, Savage A (1984) Br J Surg 71: 363-367

29.  Mosimann F, Burri B, Diserens H, Fontolliet C, Coup P, Mosimann R (1979) Scand J Gastroenterol 16: 149-152

30.  Muller-Lissner SA, Fimmel CJ, Will N, Muller-Duysing W, Hemzel F, Blum AL (1982) Gastroenterology 83: 1276-1279

31.  Orchard R, Reynolds K, Fox B, Andrews R, Parkins RA, Johnson AG (1977) Gut 18: 457-461

32. Puju S, Shuker DEG, Bishop WW, Falchuk KR, Tannenbaum SR, Thilly WG (1982) Cancer Res 42: 2601-2604

33. Reddy BS, Narisawa T, Weisberger JH, Wynder EL (1976) J Nat Cancer Inst 56: 441-442

34. Rees WDW, Garner A, Turnberg LA, Gibbons LC (1982) Gastroenterology 83: 425-440

35. Ritchie WP (1980) Ann Surg 192: 288-298

36. Roux C (1897) Rev Gynecol Chir 1: 67-122

37. Savage A, Jones S (1979) J Clin Pathol 32: 179-186

38. Schlag P, Meister H, Feyerabend G, Merkle P (1977) Langenbecks Arch Chir 344: 207-217

39. Schoon IM, Andersson H, Faxen A, Olbe L (1979) Scand J Gastroenterol 14: 969-976

40. Schrumpf E, Stadaas J, Myren J, Serck-Hanssen A, Aune S, Osnes M (1977) Lancet ii: 467-469

41. Smith GM (1914) J Med Res 30: 147-184

42. Stalsberg H, Taksdal S (1971) Lancet ii: 1175-1177

43. Tabaquchali S, Okubadejo JA, Neal G, Booth CC (1966) Proc R Soc Med 59: 1244-

44. Thomas WEG, Jackson PC, Cooper MJ, Davies ER (1984) Scand J Gastroenterol 92: 36-40

45. Watt PCH, Sloan JM, Spencer A, Kennedy TL (1983) Br Med J 287: 1410-1412

# THE FUTURE

© *Elsevier Science Publishers B.V. (Biomedical Division)*
*Gastric carcinogenesis. P.I. Reed, M.J. Hill, editors.*

# ACTIONS SUGGESTED BY GASTRIC CANCER EPIDEMIOLOGICAL STUDIES IN JAPAN

TAKESHI HIRAYAMA

Institute of Preventive Oncology, HI Bldg, 1-2 Ichigaya-Sadohara, Shinjuku-ku, Tokyo 162, Japan

## INTRODUCTION

Gastric cancer ranks top among cancers of different sites in incidence in the world for both sexes together as of 1980, the number of estimated cases being 6,694,000 (IARC, 1986-87) (1). Japan ranks top in the frequency of gastric cancer among many countries in the world, the number of deaths in 1986 being 48,266 (male; 30,127, female; 18,139). The incidence of the disease is on a downward trend in most countries. Such a tendency of decline is also striking in Japan (6,7). Studies of analytical epidemiology revealed major risk factors governing the occurrence of gastric cancer (2,8-16). The breakthrough strategy for the primary prevention of the disease was considered based on such observations.

## MATERIALS

(a) Vital statistics in Japan (1948-86) and in selected countries in the world.

(b) "Cancer Incidence in Five Continents" Vol 4 (published by IARC).

(c) National Nutrition Survey (1949-82).

(d) Results of follow-up of 265,118 adults aged 40 and above in 29 health centre districts, 1966-82, in Japan.

## RESULTS

### Recent Decline in Gastric Cancer Mortality and its Reasons

A drastic decline in gastric cancer mortality rates took place in Japan, the mortality rate adjusted to 1935 census population being 48.7 in 1958 and 26.0 in 1985 in men, and 30.0 in 1958 and 15.3 in 1985 in women (Fig 1). During 1955 to 1986, the extent of decline was most striking in age 40's, 50's and 60's where ratios of rates in 1984 to those in 1955 were around 0.50 or less (Fig 2).

Such changes are interpreted as the effect of the change in food consumption and in nutritional intake in recent years, as it is observed cross-sectionally and almost simultaneously in all age groups except age 80 and above.

A steady yearly decline in salt intake recorded in the National Nutrition Survey must have played a major role since a significant rise of gastric cancer risk was observed in daily consumers of highly salted food in several case control studies conducted by the author and others. The main reason for the recent decline in salt

210

intake must be the countrywide spread of electric refrigerators in 1955 to 1970 (Fig 3), which changed the national food preservation system drastically. The traditional way of salting for food preservaton has been replaced by a new system of "cold chain", mainly composed of freezers and electric refrigerators. Such changes also brought about a rise in per capita consumption of milk, milk products and other selected nutritional foods. Daily milk drinkers were observed to carry a lower risk of gastric cancer also through case-control studies. Thus the introduction of the electric refrigerator appears to have served at least two beneficial roles.

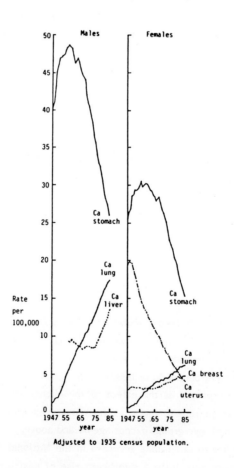

Fig. 1. Age-adjusted mortality rates for cancer of selected sites in Japan, 1947-1985.

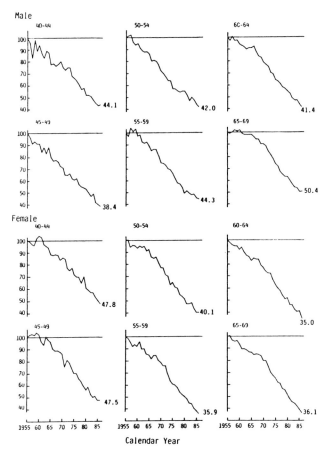

Fig. 2. Annual trend of age-specific death rate for cancer of the stomach in Japan 1955-1986 (1955 = 100).

Risk Enhancing Effect of Cigarette Smoking

Life styles of 122,261 men and 142,857 women aged 40 years and older residing in 29 Health Centre Districts were surveyed in October to December 1965 and followed up; this number represented 95% of the census population. A system of record linkage was established between original risk factor records and death certificates. Of these 5,202 (male; 3,414, female; 1,788) died of gastric cancer by the end of 1982.

A significant elevation of gastric cancer risk was observed in daily smokers compared to non-smokers. This was clearly shown by a matched group analysis where all the factors other than cigarette smoking were matched (Fig 4). The results are in line with the observations in other prospective studies in the literature (Fig 5) (17).

212

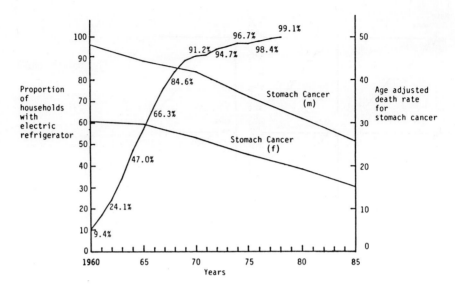

Fig. 3. Annual trends for proportion of households with electric refrigeration and age-adjusted death rates for stomach cancer in Japan, 1966-1985.

By a comparison of age cumulative mortality rate in men, it was found that the number of deaths from gastric cancer was significantly less in non-smokers than in daily smokers observed and expected deaths in non-smokers being 528 and 771.3 respectively

When a comparison was made between daily smokers and non-smokers who were 5 years older, such a difference was noted to disappear, the observed and expected deaths in non-smokers being 528 and 532.6 respectively. Therefore, the reason for the excess risk of gastric cancer in daily smokers compared with non-smokers might be due to the general tendency of 5-years ageing acceleration through daily cigarette smoking, which can be observed for many diseases other than gastric cancer (eg pancreatic cancer, ischemic heart disease), although a more specific reason such as long-term swallowing of sputum polluted by carcinogens from inhaled cigarette smoke should also be considered.

In our cohort study, daily smokers showed significantly higher standardized mortality rates for gastric cancer than non-smokers in each socio-economic strata; rates being 163.3 (per 100,000) vs 106.5 in I+II (high strata), 222.5 vs 148.6 in III, 224.4 vs 129.3 in IV and 210.3 vs 148.7 in V (lowest strata).

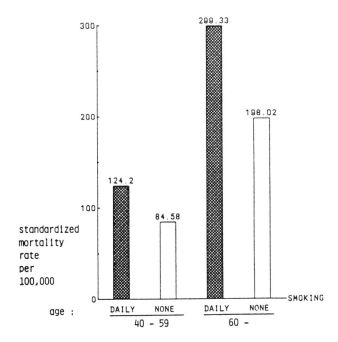

Fig. 4. Standardised mortality rate per 100,000 for cancer of the stomach by habit of cigarette smoking. A matched group analysis from the Prospective Study, Japan 1966-1981.

The risk was highest in those who started the smoking habit at an earlier age. The age standardized male mortality rates per 100,000 for those who started smoking under the age of 15, age 15-19, age 20-24, age 25-29, age 30-34, age 35 or older and non-smokers were 376.0, 238.1, 205.4, 230.4, 201.7, 151.2 and 149.0 respectively. The risk in those who had given up smoking was observed to appraoch the level of non-smokers with the lapse of years after smoking cessation; age standardized mortality rates per 100,000 being 229.3, 177.4 and 149.0 in those within 4 years after smoking cessation, 5 years or longer after smoking cessation, and non-smokers respectively.

Risk Enhancing Effect of Salted Food Intake

Daily intake of salted food was observed to enhance the risk of gastric cancer significantly by age-occupation matched case-conrol studies (Fig 6, Table 1). In males a four-fold increased risk and in females a seven-fold increased risk were noted in daily consumers of salty food compared to non-consumers in Kanagawa Prefecture (Table 1).

TABLE 1
DIET AND STOMACH CANCER : COMPARISON OF 454 CASES AND MATCHED CONTROLS (KANAGAWA PREF. 1960-61)

| | - 49 | | 50 - 59 | | 60 - | | Total | | Mantel Extension x | Standardized ratio rate |
|---|---|---|---|---|---|---|---|---|---|---|
| | S | C | S | C | S | C | S | C | | |
| **Male** | | | | | | | | | | |
| Salty food | | | | | | | | | | |
| None | 43 | 52 | 45 | 66 | 48 | 85 | 136 | 206 | | 1.000 |
| Occasional | 18 | 22 | 26 | 21 | 43 | 25 | 87 | 68 | | 1.989 |
| Daily | 22 | 9 | 27 | 11 | 28 | 9 | 77 | 29 | | 4.070 |
| Total | 83 | 83 | 98 | 98 | 119 | 119 | 300 | 300 | 6.093(p<0.0001) | |
| **Female** | | | | | | | | | | |
| Salty food | | | | | | | | | | |
| None | 30 | 38 | 19 | 43 | 13 | 34 | 62 | 115 | | 1.000 |
| Occasional | 18 | 11 | 16 | 10 | 20 | 5 | 54 | 26 | | 4.306 |
| Daily | 8 | 7 | 23 | 5 | 7 | 1 | 38 | 13 | | 7.729 |
| Total | 56 | 56 | 58 | 58 | 40 | 40 | 154 | 154 | 5.886(p<0.001) | |

S: stomach cancer;  C: control group

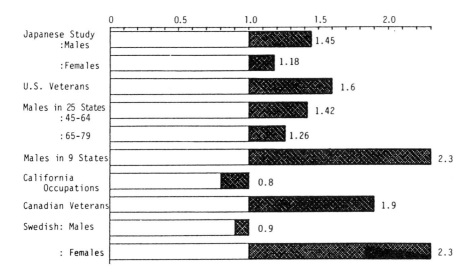

Fig. 5. Mortality ratios of current cigarette smokers for stomach cancer in seven prospective epidemiological studies.

The results are in line with the observations in other case-control studies in the literature (Fig 7) (4,5,18).

## Risk Reducing Effect of Daily Milk Intake

Daily milk intake was observed to significantly reduce the risk of gastric cancer also by the same case-control study. The risk was noted to come down to less than one fourth in males and to less than one third in females in daily milk consumers compared to non-consumers (Table 2). Such a significant trend was also observed in a large-scale cohort study described above.

## Risk Reducing Effect of Daily Green-Yellow Vegetables Intake

Daily intake of green-yellow vegetables was found to reduce the risk of gastric cancer by a large-scale cohort study conducted in 1966-82 in Japan. The standardized mortality rates for gastric cancer were observed to come down with the increase in the frequency of intake of green-yellow vegetables (Table 3).

Similar trends were observed both in males and females and in each age group (Fig 8) and both in smokers and non-smokers (Table 4, Fig 9).

The significant risk reduction was also observed in a matched group analysis where all the factors other than green-yellow vegetables consumption were matched in age 40-59 in both sexes. However, the relationship was not significant in those aged 60 and above.

TABLE 2
DIET AND STOMACH CANCER : COMPARISON OF 454 CASES AND MATCHED CONTROLS (KANAGAWA PREF. 1960-61)

| | - 49 | | 50 - 59 | | 60 - | | Total | | Mantel Extension x | Standardized ratio rate |
|---|---|---|---|---|---|---|---|---|---|---|
| | S | C | S | C | S | C | S | C | | |
| **Male** | | | | | | | | | | |
| Milk | | | | | | | | | | |
| None | 55 | 28 | 68 | 28 | 76 | 40 | 199 | 96 | | 1.000 |
| Occasional | 8 | 16 | 12 | 25 | 17 | 22 | 37 | 63 | | 0.293 |
| Daily | 20 | 39 | 18 | 45 | 26 | 57 | 64 | 141 | | 0.220 |
| Total | 83 | 83 | 98 | 98 | 119 | 119 | 300 | 300 | - 8.141(p<0.001) | |
| **Female** | | | | | | | | | | |
| Milk | | | | | | | | | | |
| None | 39 | 8 | 31 | 14 | 14 | 21 | 94 | 43 | | 1.000 |
| Occasional | 9 | 17 | 9 | 17 | 4 | 3 | 22 | 37 | | 0.422 |
| Daily | 8 | 31 | 18 | 27 | 12 | 16 | 38 | 74 | | 0.289 |
| Total | 56 | 56 | 58 | 58 | 40 | 40 | 154 | 154 | - 5.583(p<0.0001) | |

S: stomach cancer; C: control group

TABLE 3
RISK OF STOMACH CANCER BY FREQUENCY OF GREEN-YELLOW VEGETABLES CONSUMPTION - PROSPECTIVE STUDY, 1966-82, JAPAN

| Frequency of GYV Consumption | OBS/PY | Age in years | | | | | | | | Standardized Rate Ratio | Mantel-extension chi / One-tail p value |
|---|---|---|---|---|---|---|---|---|---|---|---|
| | | 40-44 | 45-49 | 50-54 | 55-59 | 60-64 | 65-69 | 70-74 | 75- | | |
| None | OBS | 0 | 1 | 0 | 1 | 2 | 5 | 7 | 1 | 1.000 | Mantel-extension chi -2.134 |
| | PY | 146 | 435 | 669 | 933 | 1001 | 970 | 724 | 506 | | |
| Rare | OBS | 0 | 0 | 3 | 12 | 13 | 18 | 21 | 16 | 0.741 | |
| | PY | 1069 | 3168 | 4938 | 6481 | 6518 | 6230 | 4601 | 3442 | | |
| Occas. | OBS | 4 | 21 | 48 | 81 | 160 | 208 | 187 | 184 | 0.707 | One-tail p value 0.01642 |
| | PY | 13996 | 40356 | 63187 | 82201 | 78243 | 70102 | 49313 | 35155 | | |
| Daily | OBS | 9 | 43 | 120 | 252 | 422 | 579 | 502 | 457 | 0.664 | |
| | PY | 36307 | 110872 | 177148 | 230883 | 221619 | 199161 | 141036 | 99912 | | |
| M None | OBS | 0 | 2 | 0 | 0 | 3 | 1 | 0 | 2 | 1.000 | Mantel-extension chi -2.551 |
| | PY | 143 | 449 | 786 | 1044 | 1073 | 977 | 756 | 615 | | |
| Rare | OBS | 0 | 1 | 6 | 2 | 10 | 3 | 10 | 6 | 0.799 | |
| | PY | 1018 | 3392 | 5498 | 7095 | 6826 | 5894 | 4185 | 3001 | | |
| Occas. | OBS | 5 | 12 | 45 | 66 | 76 | 103 | 62 | 89 | 0.720 | One-tail p value 0.00537 |
| | PY | 15523 | 48891 | 77926 | 98933 | 89778 | 75657 | 52214 | 41622 | | |
| Daily | OBS | 12 | 33 | 79 | 131 | 205 | 266 | 287 | 304 | 0.662 | |
| | PY | 45166 | 145921 | 236054 | 305666 | 283848 | 245963 | 175941 | 135351 | | |

218

TABLE 4
AGE STANDARDIZED MORTALITY RATE FOR STOMACH CANCER BY AMOUNT OF SMOKING AND BY FREQUENCY OF GREEN-YELLOW VEGETABLES CONSUMPTION (PROSPECTIVE STUDY, 1966-82, JAPAN)

| Frequency of GYV Consumption | | Amount Smoked per day | | | | Standardized Rate Ratio |
|---|---|---|---|---|---|---|
| | | Non | 1-14 | 15-24 | 25- | |
| Daily | SMR | 147.3 | 205.3 | 215.5 | 192.9 | 0.702 |
| | PY | 232237 | 365102 | 446895 | 48320 | |
| Occas. | SMR | 151.6 | 221.7 | 226.8 | 248.1 | 0.757 |
| | PY | 69657 | 131347 | 163394 | 27505 | |
| Rare | SMR | 186.7 | 172.3 | 286.7 | 231.4 | 0.798 |
| | PY | 6033 | 11195 | 12920 | 3148 | |
| None | SMR | 213.0 | 452.6 | 252.5 | 0 | 1.000 |
| | PY | 860 | 1062 | 2087 | 407 | |
| Standardized Rate Ratio | | 1.000 | 1.471 | 1.370 | | |
| Mantel-extension chi | | | Smoking | GYV | | |
| | | | 5.983 | -2.213 | | |
| one teil p value | | | $1.099 \times 10^{-9}$ | 0.01345 | | |

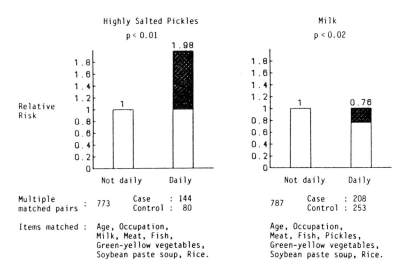

Fig. 6. Case-control study of diet and gastric cancer (The Third National Cancer Survey, 1963, Japan).

As reported before (14), those who newly became daily consumers of green-yellow vegetables during the first 6 years after the start of the cohort study still show a reduced risk of gastric cancer (Fig 10), suggesting effectiveness of dietary change after reaching adulthood.

Risk Reducing Effect of Daily Intake of Soybean Paste Soup

Soybean paste soup is one of the most popular foods in Japan. The long-term cohort study revealed a significantly lowered gastric cancer risk in daily consumers of soybean paste soup. This tendency was observed in each age group and both in smokers and non-smokers (Table 5). The significant risk reduction was also observed by a matched group analysis where all the factors other than soybean paste soup intake were matched (Table 6).

Many Japanese tend to consume soybean paste soup including green-yellow vegetables as the constitutents. Therefore, the frequency of consumption of these two food items were cross tabulated. Results showed that risk reduction by each of these was mutaually independent, the lowest risk being seen in those consuming both green and yellow vegetables (Fig 11).

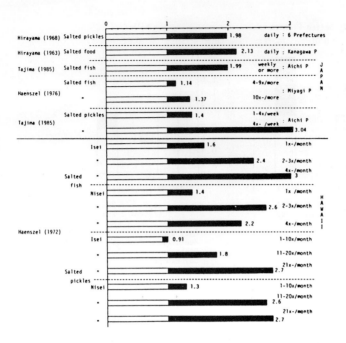

Fig. 7. Relative risk for stomach cancer in salted food consumers. Case-control studies.

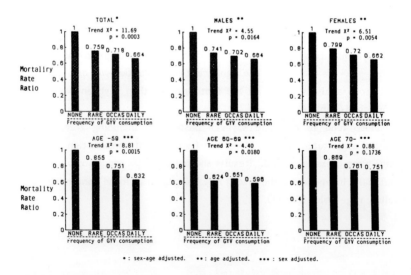

*: sex-age adjusted.   **: age adjusted.   ***: sex adjusted.

Fig. 8. Mortality rate ratio for cancer of the stomach by frequency of green-yellow vegetable consumption. Cohort study 1966-1982, Japan.

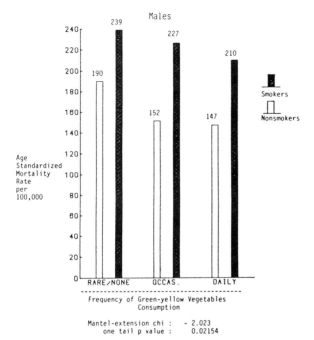

Fig. 9. Age standardised mortality rate for stomach cancer by frequency of green-yellow vegetables consumption and by smoking habit (prospective study, 1966-1982, Japan.

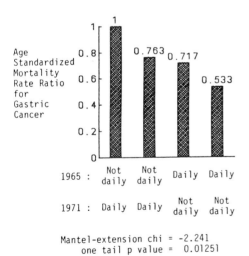

Mantel-extension chi = -2.241
one tail p value = 0.01251

Fig. 10. Changes in frequency of green-yellow vegetables consumption and subsequent mortality rate ratio for gastric cancer (age standardised) cohort study, 1971-1982, Japan (Males).

TABLE 5

STANDARDIZED MORTALITY RATE FOR CANCER OF THE STOMACH BY SMOKING AND SOYBEAN PASTE SOUP INTAKE (PROSPECTIVE STUDY, 1966-81, JAPAN)

| Cigarette | Soybean paste soup | Observed person (yr) | Standardized mortality rate (per 100,000) |
|-----------|--------------------|----------------------|-------------------------------------------|
| Male | | | |
| Daily | Daily | 860,895 | 201.4 |
| | Others | 365,237 | 242.5 |
| None | Daily | 216,656 | 133.9 |
| | Others | 78,284 | 175.4 |
| Female | | | |
| Daily | Daily | 124,751 | 87.4 |
| | Others | 83,707 | 115.2 |
| None | Daily | 1,213,245 | 81.8 |
| | Others | 504,748 | 83.3 |

| | Smoking | Soybean Paste Soup |
|---|---------|--------------------|
| Mantel-Haenszel x | 7.544 | - 4.744 |
| One-tall p-value | $2.2941 \times 10^{-14}$ | $1.0471 \times 10^{-6}$ |
| Rate ratio | 1.381 | 0.863 |
| Confidence limits | 1.287 | 0.819 |
| | 1.482 | 0.908 |

Life Styles with Highest and Lowest Risk for Gastric Cancer

In a large-scale census population-based cohort study in Japan described above, Japanese with SDA (Seventh Day Adventists)-like life styles who neither smoke cigarettes daily, nor drink alcoholic beverages daily, nor eat meat daily, but do eat green-yellow vegetables daily were found to be one of the lowest risk groups and Japanese with entirely opposite life styles, ie those who smoke, drink alcohol, and eat meat daily, but do not eat green-yellow vegetables daily were found to be the highest risk group in men (Fig 12) and in women.

TABLE 6

MATCHED GROUP ANALYSIS (MATCHED RISK FACTORS INCLUDE SEX, AGE, RESIDENCE, OCCUPATION, SMOKING, DRINKING AND DIET OTHER THAN SOYBAN PASTE SOUP)*

| | Soybean Paste Soup Intake | |
|---|---|---|
| | Daily | Not Daily |
| Number of matched pairs | 48,840 | 48,840 |
| Number of stomach cancer deaths | 799 | 932 |

$X^2 = 10.25$, p = 0.001

*Prospective study, 1966-81, Japan

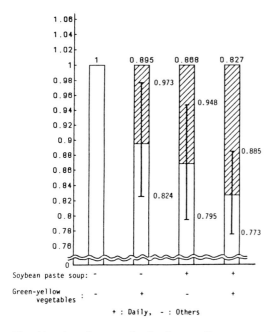

Fig. 11. Age-Sex standardised mortality rate ratio for gastric cancer by frequency of soybean paste poup consumption and green-yellow vegetables consumption (cohort study, 1966-1981, Japan)

TABLE 7

MAJOR LIFE STYLE RISK FACTORS OF GASTRIC CANCER REVEALED BY CASE-CONTROL STUDIES AND A COHORT STUDY IN JAPAN

| Type of Study | Study Area | Study Size | Major Findings |
|---|---|---|---|
| Case-Control Study | 1) Study in Kanagawa Prefectures, 1960-61 | 454 cases 454 controls matched by age, sex & occupation | Salty food    Milk |
| | 2) Study in 6 Prefectures, 1963 | 1524 cases 3792 controls matched by age, sex & occupation | Cig. smoking Highly salted pickles Milk |
| Cohort Study | 17 years follow-up (1966-82) of 265, 118 adults in 29 Health Centre Districts in 6 Prefectures | Observed person-years 3,849,637 Stomach cancer death 5,167 | Cig. smoking    Milk Green-yellow vegetables Soybean paste soup (High socio-economic strata    ) |

TABLE 8

RISK FACTORS IDENTIFIED TO ALTER GASTRIC CANCER RISK IN JAPAN

| | Traditional Risk Factors | Modern Risk Factors |
|---|---|---|
| Risk enhancing factor | Salted food | Smoking |
| Risk reducing factor | Green-yellow vegetables Soybean paste soup | Milk (Electric refrigerator) |

Japanese with SDA-opposite life styles but consuming green-yellow vegetables daily were found to have a significantly lower risk for gastric cancer compared to Japanese with SDA-opposite life styles, demonstrating again the beneficial effect of daily consumption of green-yellow vegetables in reducing gastric cancer risk (Fig 12).

Japanese with SDA-opposite life styles but who do not drink alcohol daily were also observed to show a reduced risk of gastric cancer (Fig 12).

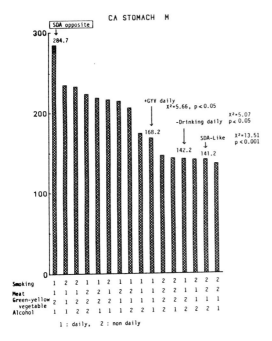

Fig. 12. Age standardised mortality rate per 100,000 by life style combination (prospective study, 1966-1981, Japan)

## ACTIONS SUGGESTED BY GASTRIC CANCER EPIDEMIOLOGIAL STUDIES

Major life style risk factors revealed by our case-control studies and a cohort study are listed in Table 7 and could be grouped into four categories, as shown in Table 8.

Apparently factors modifying the risk of gastric cancer are complex. Some of the risk factors listed in Table 8 are independent of each other while some are interrelated to each other. There are also common denominators. For instance, the introduction of electric refrigerators must have a double beneficial effect by reducing the frequency of intake of salty food and also by enhancing the consumption of milk, meat and fruits which are considered nutritious and beneficial in reducing gastric cancer risk.

These epidemiological findings strongly suggest mechanisms of gastric cancer occurrence fitting well Correa's aetiological model for gastric carcinogenesis (3) and also the currently accepted concept of multistage carcinogenesis, especially when these are viewed from the standpoint of initiator/promoter/inhibitor interaction model.

Cancer initiators and promoters are known to exist in cigarette smoke. Frequent intake of highly salted food has been postulated as having promoter-like effects. Beta-carotene, vitamin C, minerals and fibre-rich green-yellow vegetables, vitamin A and other nutrients in milk and selected chemical components of soybean (eg protease inhibitor) have been considered mostly as promoter and/or initiator inhibitors.

The observation of varying risks for gastric cancer in Japanese with different combinations of life-styles clearly demonstrate breakthrough strategies for gastric cancer primary prevention.

In particular, daily consumption of green-yellow vegetables coupled with cessation of smoking and avoidance of daily alcohol drinking were found to significantly reduce the risk for gastric cancer.

In the case of gastric cancer, existing control activities in Japan are now mostly concentrated on early detection programmes by mass screening which belong to secondary prevention. The identification of high-risk groups is of importance in order to improve the efficiency of mass screening. The above described epidemiological findings delineate characteristics of such high risk groups. However, the primary use of such epidemiological observations should be for the establishment of strategies for primary prevention which could be carried out in parallel with programmes of secondary prevention.

These strategies are all within our reach and can be carried out without much cost by well-planned intensive public education plus creative campaigns by the mass media. The effect of such an endeavour can be seen in promising changes in life styles emerging in Japan in recent years (Table 9). The well balanced integration of strategies both for primary and secondary prevention under careful consideration of cost-effectiveness must result in further rapid reduction of gastric cancer morbidity and mortality in Japan in the near future.

TABLE 9

PROMISING CHANGES IN LIFE STYLES IN JAPAN

|  |  | 1975 | 1985 |
|---|---|---|---|
| (1) Smoking rate | m | 76.2% | 62.5% |
|  | f | 15.1% | 12.6% |
| (2) Salt consumption |  | 13.5g | 12.1g |
| (3) Milk and milk products |  | 103.6g | 116.7g |
| (4) Green-yellow vegetables consumption |  | 48.2g | 73.9g |

REFERENCES

1.  Biennial Report 1986-1987 (1987) IARC, Lyon, p11

2.  Cancer Risks by Site (1980) Hirayama T, Waterhouse J, Fraumeni J (eds) UICC Technical Report series 41

3.  Correa P, Haenszel W, Cuello C, Tannenbaum S, Archer M (1975) Lancet ii:58-60

4.  Haenszel W, Kurihara N, Segi M, Lee RKC (1972) J Natl Canc Inst 49:969-988

5.  Haenszel W, Kurihara M, Locke FB, Shimizu K, Segi M (1976) 56:265-274

6.  Hirayama T (1975) Cancer Res 35:3460-3463

7.  Hirayama T (1977) In: Hiatt HH et al (eds) Origins of Human Cancer. Book A. Cold Spring Harbor Lab, Cold Spring Harbor, pp55-75

8.  Hirayama T (1963) Bull Inst Public Health 12:85-96

9.  Hirayama T (1967) In: Harris RJC (ed) UICC Monogr Series 10, Ninth International Cancer Cong. Springer - Verlag pp37-49

10. Hirayama T (1971) In: Murakami T (ed) Early Gastric Cancer. Gann Monogr on Cancer Res 11. Jpn Cancer Assoc, Tokyo, pp3-19

11. Hirayama T (1979) In: Pfeiffer CJ (ed) Gastric Cancer. Gerhard Witzstrock Publ House Inc, New York, pp60-82

12. Hirayama T (1981) In: Fielding JW et al (eds) Gastric Cancer 32. Pergamon Press, Oxford and New York, pp1-15

13. Hirayama T (1982) In: Tominaga S, Aoki K (eds) The UICC Smoking Control Workshop 1981. The University of Nagoya Press, Nagoya, pp2-8

14. Hirayama T (1982) In: Bartsch H, Armstrong B, Davis W (eds) Proceedings of Symposium on Host Factors in Human Carcinogenesis. IARC (Scientific Publication No 39), Lyon, pp531-540

15. Hirayama T (1982) Nutr and Cancer 3:223-233

16. Hirayama T (1986) In: Hayashi Y et al (eds) Diet, Nutrition and Cancer. Jpn SCI SOC Press, Tokyo/VNU SCI Press, Utrecht, pp41-53

17. Smoking and Health, A Report of the Surgeon General (1979) US Dept of Health, Education and Welfare, pp2-40

18. Tajima K, Tominaga S (1985) Gann 76:705-716

© Elsevier Science Publishers B.V. (Biomedical Division)
Gastric carcinogenesis. P.I. Reed, M.J. Hill, editors.

ECP-EURONUT INTESTINAL METAPLASIA STUDY: DESIGN OF THE STUDY WITH SPECIAL REFERENCE TO THE DEVELOPMENT AND VALIDATION OF THE QUESTIONNAIRE

C E WEST, W A van STAVEREN
Departmnet of Human Nutrition, Wageningen Agricultural University Bomenweg 2, 6703 HD Wageningen, The Netherlands

INTRODUCTION

Intestinal metaplasia is regarded as a precursor lesion of the intestinal type of stomach cancer. It has been suggested by Correa et al (4) that the first stage in the development of such cancer is the development of gastric atrophy, in which nutritional factors appear to play a role. One factor thought to be implicated in this step is dietary salt (6). Gastric atrophy results in hypochlorhydria and consequently bacterial overgrowth of the stomach. Bacteria reduce dietary nitrate to nitrite and also catalyse the subsequent N-nitrosation of suitable secondary amino groups by that nitrite; these N-nitroso compounds may be involved in the development of increasingly severe dysplasia and ultimately malignancy. The reduction of nitrate to nitrite is inhibited by vitamin C, vitamin E and selenium which can replace a part of the vitamin E requirement. This hypothesis has generated much interest but it is by no means proven. The purpose of the ECP-EURONUT intestinal metaplasia project is to examine the first step in the pathway suggested for the aetiology of the intestinal type of gastric cancer.

One of the biggest problems in trying to relate nutritional factors to cancer is that by the time cancer has been diagnosed it is difficult to determine the nature and quantity of food eaten at the critical time for the development of the cancer. This is so for a number of reasons:

Firstly, onset of the disease produces changes in eating patterns; and secondly, the critical time for cancer development, that is when cancer is initiated and during the initial stages of promotion, could be many years prior to clinical manifestation of the disease.

As intestinal metaplasia is a very important precancerous lesion, a study aimed at elucidating factors involved in the aetiology of this disease would give information on factors involved in the aetiology of gastric cancer with fewer of the problems referred to above.

The work described in this chapter was carried out within the framework of the joint intestinal metaplasia (atrophic gastritis) project of the Diet and Cancer Group of the European Organization of Cooperation in Cancer Prevention Studies (ECP) and EURONUT which is the concerted action programme of nutrition within the

European Communities (10).

## AIM OF THE STUDY

The hypothesis being tested is that there is a significant difference between cases and controls in the intake of foods, nutrients and toxicants with special emphasis being given to those which have been postulated as being associated with type B atrophic gastritis, intestinal metaplasia or with gastric carcinoma. A case-control study is being carried out involving 600 subjects in each of the countries participating in the project. As the study is being carried out in a number of European countries (Greece, Italy, Poland, Portugal, United Kingdom and Yugoslavia), those factors which are found to be associated with intestinal metaplasia in a high proportion of countries are likely to be of great importance in the aetiology of this disease and of gastric cancer.

## METHODS
### Selection of Cases and Controls

Cases are being selected from patients, aged between 20 and 55 years, attending clinics with upper gastrointestinal complaints which justify carrying out a gastric biopsy. Three good biopsies will be taken from three sites: 5 cm from the pylorus on the greater curvature, at the angulus in the antrum on the lesser curvature, and in the fundic area (fornix) of the greater curvature. Sections are to be prepared from the biopsies, stained and examined following strict guidelines with strong central supervision by Dr I Filipe in London. Those found to have intestinal metaplasia are eligible for inclusion in the study. The remainder of those undergoing gastroscopy are eligible for inclusion as the first group of controls (endoscopy controls). A second group of controls is being selected from apparently healthy persons in the population at large or, in a number of centres, from people attending other clinics such as an orthopaedic or dermatological clinic (non-endoscopy controls). Controls will be matched for age within three years, for sex and for time of year.

### Measurement of Food Intake

Much effort has been directed towards the development and validation of a method suitable for measurement of food intake in the past. The obvious method of choice is a retrospective dietary history using a questionnaire enquiring about usual food consumption in a selected period in the past and a structured food frequency list. Retrospective diet histories are impossible to validate with certainty. However, a number of studies have been carried out in various countries to assess their relative validity by interviewing people who participated in food consumption studies in the past. Data from these "initial" food consumption studies were taken as reference and compared with data from retrospective dietary interviews. In order to develop a suitable method for the intestinal metaplasia study, three validation studies were carried out in the Netherlands.

In the first validation study, 79 adults were interviewed by use of the dietary history method about their intake four years previously. These results were compared with those obtained in the same group by means of a seven-day record method four years earlier. The results of the study were considered to be satisfactory (8) but, because the original data were obtained by a seven-day record method and in the retrospective study a dietary history method was employed, methodological differences may have accounted for some disagreement.

In the second validation study, a retrospective dietary history was compared with a dietary history taken seven years previously. In addition, the current intake was measured by means of a second dietary history. By so doing it was hoped to establish whether present intake, or the degree of change in the dietary intake, influences the responses in the retrospective dietary interviewing. Ninety-one adults participated in this study. The difference found between the intake assessed contemporaneously and retrospectively appeared to be the same as in our first study. This was disappointing because we had expected that the correspondence between the two estimates would have been improved because of the better study design employed in the second study. The lack of improvement may have been due to the difference in time interval of seven years as distinct from the earlier study which referred to a period four years previously. The results of the second study suggest that the currently assessed intake of food at the present time gives as good an indication of food intake in the past as does a current assessment of past food intake (9). Other investigators (1,7) have also concluded that a more valid method of assessing food consumption retrospectively may be found if more attention is paid to changes in food consumption occurring over the time period in question.

In the third validation study, we examined whether the food frequency method would be useful in monitoring major changes in food intake over long periods of time. This approach was evaluated in a study of two groups of apparently healthy elderly people who had participated in a food consumption study 12-14 years previously (1). One group comprised 18 harbour employees who had retired subsequent to the initial assessment of food intake. This group had reduced their daily food consumption by about 1000 KJ on average. The other group comprised 46 elderly men and women, who had retired before their food consumption was measured initially. The results showed that both groups overestimated changes in their food intake and that the systematic overestimation and random error were similar for both groups. In this study, changes in food intake within each group of subjects were very similar and the spread in energy and nutrient intake was low. If the intake of food or nutrients is related to a disease, the study population is expected to have a large spread in intake of energy and the various nutrients. Low spread would indicate a small difference in exposure to a risk factor between cases and controls and this is unlikely. Thus in order to obtain not only a larger but also a more realistic group of subjects from an epidemiological point of view, the males in both groups of subjects were combined to form a new group. This combined group was less homogeneous with respect to the changes in food intake and to absolute energy and nutrient intake. The agreement between the assessment of energy and nutrient intake of the original and retrospective dietary histories were better for the combined group than for the two groups separately. As expected, the degree of misclassification into small, medium and large consumers was lower in this combined group.

These three validation studies clearly show that for studies on the role of nutritional factors in the onset of a disease with a long latency time such as intestinal metaplasia or gastric cancer itself, it is possible to collect retrospective data rather than current data. This enables changes in diet to be taken into account. However, the results have shown that current diet affects retrospective reporting and that it is hard to develop a method which can correct for this effect (see also ref 3). The method developed for the study involves measuring the present food intake using a dietary history with a time frame of one months. In addition, changes in food intake which have occurred since the age of 30 years (25 years for subjects younger than 30 years) are assessed using a food frequency method. The method was tested in a series of pilot studies and the results were discussed at a workshop held in Wageningen in May 1986.

Measurement of Intake of Nutrients and Other Substances

In the measurement of food intake, special attention is being directed towards the measurement of intake of nutrients and toxicants thought to be related to the aetiology of either intestinal metapalsia or to gastric cancer itself. These include the following:

- energy, protein, fat, dietary fibre and alcohol,
- vitamin A, carotenes, vitamin C and iron,
- foods containing N-nitroso compounds such as salted and smoked meat and fish products,
- foods containing secondary amines such as salted and smoked meat and fish products, salted and pickled vegetables, and
- foods containing nitrite such as preserved meat, potatoes, other vegetables and spiced foods.

Since data on food consumption will be collected from more than one country in Europe, it is essential that the food composition tables are compatible. Thus, there will be great reliance on the work of the EUROFOODS organization which has been established to do just this (5). Intake of electrolytes, nitrite, and a number of other substances will be estimated by analysis of 24-hour urine samples. In some centres, p-aminobenzoic acid (PABA) will also be measured in urine after ingestion of PABA to measure completeness of urine collection. The nitrate analyses will be carried out at the Bacterial Metabolism Research Laboratory of the Centre for Applied Microbiology and Research at Porton Down (England).

Other Determinations

In some centres, other parameters will be measured. For example, to examine the role of Campylobacter pylori in the aetiology of intestinal metaplasia, antibodies to this bacterium are being measured in blood. Pepsinogens I and II and gastrin will be measured in some centres to evaluate their use in the diagnosis of intestinal metaplasia. In addition some centres will collect blood for the determination of serum for vitamin A, beta-carotene, vitamin C, vitamin E and selenium.

CONCLUSIONS

It is expected that collection of data will be completed in the United Kingdom, Poland and Italy by the end of 1988 and in Greece, Portugal and Yugoslavia before the end of 1989.

Preliminary results are just starting to come in from the various centres but it will take some time before the stage is reached when all statistical analyses are complete. If the hypothesis that certain foods and nutrients are related to the aetiology of intestinal metaplasia proves to be correct, the next step will be to examine more closely the relationship between diet and the progression from intestinal metaplasia to gastric cancer.

REFERENCES
1. Bakkum A, Bloemberg B, Van Staveren WA, Verschuren M, West CE (1988) Nutr Cancer 11:41-53
2. Byers TE, Rosenthal RI, Marshall JR, Rzepka TF, Cummings KM, Graham S (1983) Nutr Cancer 5:69-77
3. Byers TE, Haughey BP, Marshall JR, Swanson MK (1987) Am J epidemiol 125:351-363
4. Correa P, Haenszel W, Cuello C, Tannenbaum S, Archer M (1975) Lancet ii:58-60
5. EUROFOODS: Towards compatibility of nutrient data banks in Europe (1985) West CE (ed) Ann Nutr Metab 29, supplement 1:1-72
6. Joossens JV, Geboers J (1980) Nutr Cancer 2:251-261
7. Moller Jensen O, Wahrendorf J, Rosenqvist A, Geser A (1984) Am J epidemiol 120:281-290
8. Van Leeuwen FE, De Vet HCW, Hayes RB, Van Staveren WA, West CE,

Hautvast JCAJ (1983) Am J epidemiol 118:752-758

9.  Van Staveren WA, West CE, Hoffmans MDAF, Bos P, Kardinal AFM, Van Poppel GAFC, Schipper HJA, Hautvast JGAJ, Hayes RB (1986) Am J epidemiol 123:884-93

10. West CE (1985) EURO-NUT Report 4. Wageningen; NIVV

© Elsevier Science Publishers B.V. (Biomedical Division)
Gastric carcinogenesis. P.I. Reed, M.J. Hill, editors.

EARLY DETECTION OF GASTRIC CANCER AND PRECURSOR LESIONS

JOHANNES MYREN
Deparment of Gastroenterology, Ulleval Hospital, Oslo 4, Norway

INCIDENCE AND MORTALITY OF GASTRIC CANCER

The incidence rates of gastric cancer (1,6,18,24,47) have varied in different countries and from time to time. In 1958-62 the incidence per million inhabitants in Japan was 1610 for males and 846 for females compared to 510 for males and 305 for females in Europe and 380 for males and 250 for females in other parts of the World. In 1973-82 the incidence had decreased by 14% for males and 18% for females in Japan, whereas in Europe the decrease was 50% both for men and women, and in other parts of the world 30% for men and 50% for women.

The mortality of gastric cancer which in the same year periods was about two thirds of the incidence rate, has shown similar variations. It is well known that the 5-year survival of patients with advanced gastric cancer is very poor and recently reported to be on average 12.5% (5-65%),highly dependent on the size and location of the malignancy, and the progression beyond the submucosal layers of the stomach (46). The decrease in mortality during the last two decades has partly been ascribed to a lowering of the incidence of the intestinal type which has a higher mortality than the diffuse type (18), improvement of living conditions and therapeutic procedures (46).

The improvements in detection of carcinomas confined to the gastric mucosa (early gastric cancer) has given new hope for the future (7,26,40,52,54,56,58,61,63). In Japan the introduction of the gastrocamera and fiberoptic endoscopic methods for mass screening resulted in detection of up to 40% of the malignancies as early cancer. In Europe and North America with a lower incidence of gastric cancer, 6-10% have been diagnosed in the early stage. At Ulleval Hospital early gastric cancer was diagnosed in 12% of patients with malignancies of the stomach in 1971-75 compared to 17% in the years 1976-80 parallel to the increase in number of gastroscopies performed (52,54,56,61,63). During this period early gastric cancer accounted for 27% of malignancies found in patients operated previously for benign peptic ulcer (63). The varying rates of detection may partly depend on difficulties in identifying the Japanese depressed type IIc of early cancer which may be diagnosed as peptic ulcer (7).

Following the rapid expansion of fiberoptic endoscopic methods including cytology and bioptic histology precursor conditions and lesions were defined more precisely than before (1,2,3,11,18,25,34,37,48,50,53,54,56,57,58,61,63,65).

## THE PRECURSOR CONDITIONS

The resected stomach more than 10 years previously for a peptic ulcer was found by many investigators to be associated with a 3-6 fold increase in risk for stump carcinoma in relation to the general population at the same age (11,18,26,48,54,56,61,63). An increased risk for gastric cancer was also observed in patients with pernicious anemia, adenomatous polyps of the stomach, Menetriers disease and gastric ulcer.

Members of families with a high incidence of gastric cancer and patients with chronic gastritis were also found to have an increased risk for malignancy of the stomach (11,25,48,50). An increased incidence of gastric cancer was also observed in populations living on diet rich in fish and vitamin A (53).

## THE PRECURSOR LESIONS

The significant histological finding in endoscopic biopsies showing gastric mucosal epithelial disorganization is dysplasia (11,48,50), which has been graded as mild (I), moderate (II) and severe (III). The incidence in patients subjected to gastroscopy has been found to be 5-6% for I, 3-4% for II and 1-2% for III (cancer-in-situ), representing a definite high risk precursor lesion (19,48,50,71). The Grades I and II dysplasia cannot easily be discriminated from regenerative changes. In patients with a previous partial gastrectomy for peptic ulcer, atrophic gastritis has been found in 50-100%, mild and moderate dysplasia in 15-60% and severe dysplasia in 3% (2,3,54,61).

## EARLY DETECTION OF CANCER

Mass screening with double contrast X-ray and endoscopic methods has been performed with excellent results in Japan, where the incidence of gastric carcinoma is three times as high as in Western countries (18,21,26,40). Therefore, in these countries examination of large populations would represent an unacceptable cost per detected cancer. Early detection of malignant lesions will thus depend on screening procedures of patients with precursor conditions or symptoms and clinical and laboratory findings suspicious of carcinoma.

The value of symptoms and routine clinical and laboratory examinations (10,29,32,51). Examination of symptoms by questionnaires and interviews (10,29) showed that significant discriminants for advanced carcinoma of the stomach were reduced appetite, weight loss, food sticking and nausea in 25-65% of cases only. The five years survival in these patients was, however, poor (15%) even if the duration of the symptoms was less than 3 months. Palpation of a tumour was a late finding, and blood in stool and anemia were absent in most of the patients even with advanced carcinoma (16). A systematic healthy control study in Japan including programmed registration of symptoms and laboratory tests showed, however, a detection rate superior to that in conventional outpatients clinics.

Hartley et al (30) examined 30 patients with early gastric cancer in comparison to 278 with advanced carcinomas. In the group with early cancer the mean age (62.9 years for men and 60.7 years for women) was significantly lower than for the group with advanced carcinoma (67.3 and 70.9 years, respectively). Complaints of pain were found in 63% of patients with early gastric cancer and 60% of cases with advanced carcinoma, the symptoms being present for less than half a year in 83% and 81%, respectively. Weight loss was observed in 37% and 60%, anorexia in 23% and 55% in the cases with early and advanced cancer, respectively. The mean blood concentration of haemoglobin at the time of diagnosis was similar in both groups, about 12 g/100 ml. The occurrence of the blood group A was 27% in patients with early cancer compared to 47% in those with advanced cancrcinoma.

The value of specialized laboratory tests (4,5,8,12,17,20,22,36,59,64,65,67,68). Authors agree that determinations of carcinoembryonic antigen (CEA), CA12-5, CA19-9, CA50 and alpha foetoprotein show a low sensitivity in the early detection of gastric cancer, although they may be useful int he follow-up of recurrences after surgical intervention (10,13,18,34). Also measurements of muco-glucoproteins in gastric juice and immunohistochemical markers for serotonin, gastrin, somatostatin and beta-human chorionic gonadotrophin have shown a low sensitivity. The oncogene expression transforming gene of the human DNA has attracted much attention, but is still without practical application.

Determination of gastric enzymes as a screening test for gastric cancer was studied by Finch et al (22) in gastric washings from 445 patients submitted for routine endoscopy. Out of the 24 patients with gastric carcinoma 21 had elevated values for lactic dehydrogenase and beta-glucuronidase including four with early carcinoma.

The Value of Radiological and Endoscopic Methods

Although a similar accuracy has been reported between biphasic radiology and fiberoptic endoscopy in differentiation between peptic ulcer and gastric cancer (64), authors agree that the endoscopic methods show higher detection rates for early gastric cancer than X-ray examinations using double contrast media (11,14,15,18,19,21,23,27,28,30,31,33,41,43, 44,45,46,62,67,72).

Takasu et al (67) studied 910 matched Japanese pairs of patients and found a similar sensitivity by the radiologial and endoscopic methods (86% and 80%, respectively). But the percent false positive tests were significantly higher by the radiologic than by the endoscopic method (69% and 17%, respectively). In this study all overlooked gastric cancers were in the proximal part of the stomach where supplementary methods are needed.

Hartley et al (30) studied 30 cases of early gastric cancer out of a series of 308 with carcinoma of the stomach (9.7%). The detection rates for the two methods at the first examination was 69% for endoscopy and 40% for X-ray examination. Similar results were found in a recent series of 64 patients of early gastric cancer and in 17 out of 302 cases of carcinoma of the stomach, all with dyspeptic symptoms.

In the proximal part of the stomach where endoscopy with biopsy fails more than in the distal part, double contrast radiology has been recommended as a supplement to endoscopic guided multiple biopsies (18). In 51 patients with carcinoma of the lower oesophagus and cardia Lusink et al (45) found the larger biopsies obtained by the rigid endoscope superior to the smaller biopsies by the flexible gastroscope.

In recent years great interest has been given to endoscopic ultrasonography (60,70). A high degree of accuracy has been found in the estimation of the extent of malignant infiltraton of 62 cases of oesophageal and gastric carcinomas as an indicator of resectability (70). Great interest has also been focused on magnetic resonance imaging for the determination of the extent and operability of diffusely infiltrating malignancies (73). The final answer to these problems has not yet been given.

Endoscopy with multiple biopsies should be performed in all patients suspected of malignancy of the stomach. In 1972-1982 the results of pre-operative fiberoptic biopsy examination in 771 patients with early carcinoma were compared by Itabashi et al (35) to the histology of the resected specimens. At the initial histology of the biopsies a correct diagnosis was obtained in 87%. Repeated endoscopy with biopsies in the failures resulted in a correct diagnosis in 96%. The false negative diagnoses were mainly due to difficult differentiation from regenerative atypia in cases with the Japanese type IIc (depressed) lesions, and from adenomatous polyps in patients with elevated lesions.

Serck-Hanssen (63) studied 43 cases of early gastric cancer out of 467 with carcinoma of the stomach (9.2%) and found that the ratio of histologic diagnoses positive for cancer increased from 43% to 85% when the number of biopsies was increased from 2-4 to 16-20. This was particularly demonstrated in 10 cases of early carcinoma among a total of 70 cases of malignancies from the resected stomach for benign peptic ulcer (18%). The routine at Ulleval Hospital has since then been to take 20 biopsies from the operated stomach irrespective of endoscopic findings as stressed by Schrumpf et al (61). By this method advanced carcinoma was detected in 3 patients, early carcinoma in one and severe dysplasia in 3 of 108 patients operated 14 years previously for duodenal ulcer with BII partial gastrectomy.

Previous observations of the increased occurrence of malignant and precursor lesions in the gastric remnant (15,43,54,61) have recently been confirmed by Offerhaus et al (54) in 504 patients 24 years after partial gastrectomy and by Greene et al (28) in 163 patients operated upon 14.6 years previously for benign peptic ulcers. In both studies 1.8% of the patients had adenocarcinoma. In 50% early carcinoma was detected, some of which were not visible by endoscopy.

In general endoscopy with multiple biopsies provides a correct diagnosis in 90-95% of cases (2,27,35,38,42,45,50,62). In cases with results for malignancy which are negative but still suspicious, re-examination should be performed within a few days to one month, particularly if histology shows severe dysplasia (11,25,48,50,54,56,61,63). Special care should be given to patients with strictures and retention of content in whom a false negative result may be obtained (57).

The importance of cytology has been reviewed by Chambers and Clark (9) in 1157 samples from an 8-year period and compared to the results of biopsy. Cytology was reported to be positive in 85% of 225 cases of malignancy with three false positive diagnoses (0.3%), whereas suspicious findings for carcinoma were found in 5%. In half of these cases a final diagnosis of malignancy was made. Histology alone detected malignancy in 90.2%, whereas a combination of cytology and histology on biopsy proved correct in 95.7%. A similar increased accuracy by combining endoscopic biopsy and cytology was found by Morena-Otero (49) in 194 proven cases of cancer, in which cytology alone provided 90% correct diagnoss and biopsy 79% and by Young et al (74).

## EARLY DIAGNOSIS OF PRECURSOR CONDITIONS

(a) Patients with previous gastrectomy for benign peptic ulcers. An increased incidence of cancer and precursor lesions has been reported 10 years and more after the partial gastrectomy by several authors (54,61). A follow-up programme including endoscopy with multiple biopsies is recommended. The frequency of re-examinations depends mainly on the histological findings of severe dysplasia.

(b) Patients with gastric polyps. Polypectomy should be performed, and re-examinations performed according to the histological findings.

(c) Patients with chronic gastritis, pernicious anemia, gastric ulcers and Menetriers disease. Re-examinations with endoscopic methods including multiple biopsies, supplemented with cytology and staining methods will depend on histological findings of dysplasia.

## EARLY DIAGNOSIS OF PRECURSOR LESIONS

Significant diagnostic value of clinical symptoms, findings and conventional laboratory tests seem not to be shown and a reliable sensitivity and specificity of the special laboratory tests (see earlier in this chapter), has not been demonstrated

(5,17).

Endoscopy with muliple biopsies is considered the most reliable method for demonstration of atrophic gastritis without and with intestinal metaplasia, and dysplasia. Multiple biopsies should be obtained from all areas of the stomach.

The value of endoscopic staining methods has mainly been studied in Japan where a high percentage of early cancer has been found (66,69). Staining of the gastric mucosa has been performed by direct spraying through the gastroscope with a solution of 0.5% methylene blue under direct vision. Two minutes later the dye is washed out with distilled water and the lesions are visualized by blue color. Staining may also be obtained with peroral administrtion of a capsule containing the dye, mucus being removed by giving a proteolytic solution. About 90% correct diagnosis of early gastric cancer may be obtained by this method (66). Tatsuta et al (69) studying 761 patients with early gastric cancer, found that staining of the mucosa in the upper part of the stomach with Congo red and methylene blue improved the accuracy of diagnosis from 27% by endoscopy and biopsy to 75-83% when staining was added.

No satisfactory controlled study seems yet to be published, and in the Western world the evidence is scanty.

COMMENTS AND CONCLUSIONS

Improvement of the poor prognosis of patients with gastric cancer may be obtained by improving our knowledge and surveillance of subjects with precursor conditions. Optimal screening and examination methods should be agreed upon for detection of precursor lesions and early gastric cancer. Of high importance is also an acceptable programme for surveillance. aims for the future may be:

Establishing an international programme for mapping of patients with precursor conditions, coordinated by the OMGE.

Establishing an international programme for examination and follow-up of patients wih precursor lesions and early gastric cancer.

Cooperative studies of the best endoscopic-radiological methods. At the present time the endoscopic methods are the most profitable.

Patients with negative results but still suspicious of a malignancy should be re-examined as soon as possible with cytology and or a staining method in addition to endoscopy with multiple biopsies.

Patients with severe dysplasia should be re-examined at short intervals if no contraindications are found.

Patients with mild and moderate dysplasia may be re-examined at 3-5 years intervals should a therapeutic procedure be profitable.

REFERENCES

1. Alum WH (1986) Br Med J 293 (6546):541-543

2. Andersson A, Lauritsen KB, West F, Johansen AA (1987) Acta Chir Scand 153:29-31

3. Aste H, Sciallero S, Pugliese V, Gennaro M (1986) Endoscopy 18:174-176

4. Bassalyk LS, Ljubimova NV (1987) Neoplasma 34:319-324

5. Bazuro GE, Koch M, Cimmino G, Poti GP, Cava MC, Capurso L (1986) Endoscopy 9:45

6. Berndt H, Neumann P (1983) Z aertzl Fortbild 77:16-20

7. Blackstone MO (1984) Gastrointest Endoscopy 30:105-106

8. Borch K, Lundin C, Sahren B (1987) Gut 25:26-37

9. Chambers LA, Clark WE (1986) Acta Cytol (Baltimore) 30:110-114

10. Chisholm EM, Marshall RJ, Brown D, Cooper EH, Giles GR (1986) Br J Cancer 53:53-57

11. Correa P (1982) Cancer 50:2554-2565

12. Correa P, Montes G, Cuello C, Haenszel W, Liuzza G, Zaramo G, de Marin E, Zavala D (1985) Natl Cancer Inst Monogr 69:121-123

13. de Dombal FT, Unwin BJ, Cotton P, Giles GR, Morgan AG, Price AB, Thompson H, Williams GT (1986) Digest Dis Sci 31 Suppl:219S

14. Doebroente Z, Karaczony G, Nafradi J, Pap A, Varro V (1980) Wien Klin Wschr 92:118-122

15. Domellof L, Erikson S, Janunger KG (1977) Gastroenterology 73:462-468

16. Dybdahl JH (1984) Scand J Gastroenterol 19:1-10

17. Dykes PW, Bradwell AR (1987) GI Futures 2:12-14

18. Elder JB (1987) Curr Opin Gastroenterol 3:1015-1025

19. Evans E, Harris O, Dickey D, Hartley L (1985) Aust NZ J Surg 55:541-544

20. Extor N, Dixon MF (1986) Histopathology 10:1271-1277

21. Fielding J, Ellis D, Jones B et al (1981) Br Med J 281:985-987

22. Finch PJ, Ryan FP, Rogers K, Holt S (1987) Gut 28:319-322

23. Gaisberg von U, Femauer B (1986) Dtsch Med Wschr 111:1165-1167

24. Geboers JEF, Joossens JV, Kesteloot H (1985) Int Congr Series 685:81-95

25. Geboers K, Desmet VJ (1983) Acta Gastroenterol Belg 46:556-566

26. Goldstein F, Kline TS, Kline IK, Thornton JJ, Abrahamson J, Bell L (1983) Amer J Gastroenterol 78:715-719

27. Green PHR, O'Toole KM, Weinberg LM, Goldfarb JP (1981) Gastroenterology 81:247-257

28. Greene FL (1987) Arch Surg 122:300-303

29. Gutz H-J (1983) Z Aertzl Fortbild 77:546-549

30. Hartley L, Evans E, Dickey D, Deth A van (1983) Aust NZ J Surg 55:341-346

31. Heyder N, Lux G (1986) Scand J Gastroenterol 21 Suppl 123:47-51

32. Hinohara S, Takahashi T, Suzuki S (1983) Med Inform (Lond) 8:89-93

33. Ichikawa H (1976) In: Bostroem H et al (ed) Health control in detection of

cancer. Almquist & Wicksell, Stockholm, pp276-291

34. Ihamaeki T, Kekki M, Sipponen P, Siurala M (1985) Scand J Gastroenterol 20:485-490

35. Itabashi M, Hirota T, Unakami M, Uneo M, Oguro Y, Yamada T, Kitaoka H, Ichikawa H (1984) Jpn J Clin Oncol 14:253-270

36. Iwamatsu M, Saito T, Matsuguchi T, Tamada R, Soeijma K, Inokuchi K (1980) Cell Mol Biol 26:287-291

37. Jacobasch KH, Gutz H-J, Reitzig P (1981) Arch Geschwulstforsch 51:705-712

38. Jorde R, Ostensen H, Bostad LH, Burhol PG, Langmark FT (1986) Cancer 58:376-382

39. Kasugai T, Kobayashi S (1974) Gastroenterol 62:199-205

40. Kawai K (1971) Gann Monographs Cancer Res 11:273

41. Kiil J, Andersen D (1980) Scand J Gastroenterol 15:39-45

42. Kiil J, Andersen D, Myhre Jensen O (1979) Scand J Gastroenterol 14:189-191

43. Logan R, Langman M (1983) Lancet 2:667-669

44. Longo WE, Zucker KA, Ballantyne GH, Cambria RP, Modlin IM (1987) Arch Surg 122:292-295

45. Lusink C, Sali A, Chou ST (1983) Aust NZ J Surg 83:545-549

46. McBride CM, Boddie AW (1987) South Med J 80:283-286

47. Meyers WC, Damiano RJ Jr, Rotolo FS, Postlethwait RW (1987) Ann surg 205:1-8

48. Ming S-C, Bajtai A, Correa P, Elster K, Jarvi OH, Munoz N, Nagayo T, Stemmermann GN (1984) Cancer 54:1794-1801

49. Morena-Otero R, Cantero J (1983) Acta Cytol (Baltimore) 27:485-488

50. Morson BC, Sobin LH, Grundmann E, Johansen A, Nagayo T, Serck-Hanssen A (1980) J Clin Pathol 33:711-731

51. Myren J (1972) T Norske Laegeforen 92:1674-1676

52. Myren J, Serck-Hanssen A, Marcussen J (1979) Front Gastrointest Rest 5:149-151

53. Nomura A, Yamakawa H, Ishidate T, Kamiyama S, Masuda H, Stemmermann GN, Heilbrun LK, Hankin JH (1982) J Natl Cancer Inst 68:401-405

54. Offerhaus G, Stadt J vd, Huibregtse K, Tytgat GNJ (1984) J Clin Pathol 37:748-754

55. Oiwa T, Mori M, Sugimachi K, Enjoji M (1986) J Surg Oncol 33:170-175

56. Ones M, Lotveit T, Myren J, Serck-Hanssen A (1977)

57. Pickford JR, Craven JL, Hall R, Stone WD (1984) Gut 25:393-397

58. Potet F (1977) Gastroenterol Clin Biol 1:313-318

59. Quentmeyer A, Schlag P, Geisen HP, Schmidt-Gayk H (1986) Med Klinik 8:199-201

60. Schneider K, Dickerhoff R, Bertele RM (1986) Pediatr Radiol 16:69-70

61. Schrumpf E, Serck-Hanssen A, Stadas J, Aune S, Myren J, Osnes, M (1977) Lancet 2:467-469

62. Seifert E, Butke H, Gall K, Elster K, Cote S (1979) Am J Gastroenterol 71:563-567

63. Serck-Hanssen A (1979) Scand J Gastroenterol 13 Suppl 54:106-110

64. Shaw PC, van Romunde LKJ, Griffionen G, Janssens AR, Kreuning J, Ellers GAM (1987) Radiology 163:39-42

65. Siurala M, Samloff IM, Varis K, Ihamaeki T (1977) Scand J Gastroenterol 12 Suppl 45:98-102

66. Suzuki S, Murakami H, suzuki H, Sakakibara N, Endo M, Nakayama K (1979) Int Adv Surg Oncol 2:223-241

67. Takasu S, Tsuchiya H, Kitamura A, Yoshida S, Ito M, Sakarai Y, Funatomi T, Ikegami F (1984) Jpn J Clin Oncol 14:243-252

68. Tamada R, Hiramoto Y, Nouzuka T, Okamura T, Masuda H, Kano T, Kumashiro R, Inokuchi K (1982) Jpn Surg 12:429-433

69. Tatsuta H, Okuda IS, Taniguchi H (1984) Endoscopy 16:131-134

70. Tio TL, Jager H, Tijtgat GNJ (1986) Gastroenterology 91:401-408

71. Tomatis HP, Carreno C, Bossa H, Piva A (1984) Leber-Magen-Darm 14:150-154

72. Traedgaardh B, Wehlin L, Lindstroem C (1980) Acta Chir Scand 146:357-362

73. Winkler ML, Hricak H, Higgins CB (1987) J Comp Ass Tomography 11:337-339

© *Elsevier Science Publishers B.V. (Biomedical Division)*
*Gastric carcinogenesis. P.I. Reed, M.J. Hill, editors.*

ISSUES IN THE DESIGN OF RANDOMIZED INTERVENTION TRIALS FOR GASTRIC
CANCER PREVENTION

SYLVAN B GREEN

Clinical and Diagnostic Trials Section, Biometry branch, Division of Cancer
Prevention and Control, National Cancer Institute, Bethesda, MD 20892-4200 USA

INTRODUCTION

Epidemiological studies have provided a number of leads (4) regarding the role of
diet in gastric cancer, particularly for the intestinal type. Although this cancer has
been declining in incidence, it remains the leading cancer worldwide (5). Therefore,
there is interest in intervention studies to prevent this disease. This chapter
addresses issues relevant to such studies. The first part considers the differences
between observational (epidemiological) studies and randomized intervention trials.
Then, given the decision to do a randomized trial, there is the need for proper design
(3). In my opinion, the basic requirements of design hold for all intervention trials;
however, some problems are particularly relevant for cancer prevention trials. In
addition to general principles, the specifics of gastric carcinogenesis will determine
the sensible designs of trials to prevent this disease.

For much of this chapter reference will be made to dietary intervention trials in
general, without distinguishing between macronutrients and micronutrients.
Specifically, the administration of micronutrients in pill form (as dietary
supplements) will be considered as one type of "dietary" trial. However, there are
practical considerations (eg compliance, cost) which may be quite different
depending on the nature of the intervention.

OBSERVATIONAL STUDIES AND RANDOMIZED TRIALS

Interpretation of observational studies in epidemiology is complicated by the
effects of confounding factors. In the "natural experiments" that we observe,
individuals who differ with respect to other factors that affect the risk of
developing the disease. In a randomized trial, by definition the groups are balanced
on average with respect to other risk factors, both those we know about or at least
suspect, and those that we either have not identified or are unable to measure.

In epidemiological studies of dietary factors, a particularly important problem is
the inability to measure accurately the true long-term dietary intake of the study
subjects. This is due to difficulties in measurement (eg errors in recall) and also to
fluctuations over time (eg differences between a short-term food record and
average long-term intake). In retrospective, case-control studies, there is also the
problem that the disease itself (or its precursor lesions) may influence current diet

or may bias recall of past dietary habits. In a randomized trial, an intervention is specifically administered to one group and compared to a different intervention (or no intervention) in a comparison (or control group), and differences in outcome are observed.

The argument can be raised that measurement error in dietary variables is relevant to an intervention study also, because the extent of compliance in a trial may be difficult to assess. However, the advantage of the randomized trial remains. If a reasonable degree of compliance is achieved, then the groups do differ with respect to some dietary component(s), and if such intervention is relevant to risk, a properly designed trial should be able to detect it. Furthermore, if the intervention has been properly implemented, then the study measures what we can realistically expect to achieve with a dietary manipulation, regardless of our ability to measure compliance. Of course, if the intervention is such that we can measure compliance, then we can analyse the relation between the difference in dietary intake actually achieved and the observed difference in outcome. Such considerations demonstrate the importance of proper study design. For example, as will be discussed further below, the sample size must be adequate to detect a difference that can realistically be expected in the absence of perfect compliance.

## DESIGN OF RANDOMIZED TRIALS
### Choose the Intervention

It is obvious that a trial is only as good as the intervention being investigated. What is open to some debate is how much epidemiological and laboratory evidence concerning the effect of a specific dietary factor on risk of cancer is required to justify the cost of an intervention trial. Of all cancer types, gastric cancer is certainly a good candidate for dietary intervention, but not all investigators would agree on the components of dietary intake best suited for intervention.

One alternative to choosing a single component is the "best shot" diet; the intervention consists of the best diet that a consensus of investigators would recommend. The goal of this approach, which I find quite appealing, is to maximmize the chance that a beneficial effect will be observed (and to quantify the benefit that is so achieved). A negative result in such a study, if well-designed and well-implemented, would suggest that this is not a fruitful approach to attacking this disease. However, a positive result would demonstrate clearly the value of controlling this type of cancer through prevention. Future research could then focus on identifying the important components. Some may even argue that, if one identifies a diet that reduces gastric cancer risk, there is nothing wrong with including dietary changes that, although ineffective in reducing gastric cancer, produce no harm and may even be beneficial for other conditions. However, I suspect that most would want to investigate further the basis for a positive result. At the same time, we could immediately accelerate the reduction in this disease that has already been occurring.

Another alternative is a factorial design (2), wherein more than one intervention is studied simultaneously. For example, two interventions could be studied using four groups: one-fourth of the subjects get neither intervention, one-fourth each get one of the factors alone, and one-fourth get both. An actual example relevant to the present topic is the factorial design studying micronutrients for the prevention of oesophageal cancer which has been constructed for use in a Chinese province (1).

In addition to choosing interventions on the basis of possible efficacy, the ability to achieve the intervention must also be considered. The distinction mentioned above between dietary change and micronutrient supplentation is relevant here. Another distinction is removing or decreasing a (harmful) component of the diet versus adding or increasing a (beneficial) component. The feasibility of implementing an intervention successfully in a particular location or among a particular population may determine the success of the trial.

Defining the Eligible Subjects

After deciding what the intervention is, the next decision involves who is eligible to receive it. One aspect of this is the geographic population. This is in part related to the choice of intervention. Some dietary interventions are more likely to be applicable generally (eg increasing fruits and vegetables). Other interventions are more geographically specific (eg decreasing consumption of fava beans or smoked fish). If the latter appraoch is pursued, the question arises whether there are adequate data to support such relationships; that is, be careful of chance associations seen in a single study.

Another aspect of eligibility is the age range of subjects. Harmful components of the diet may act at younger ages; it may be too late to intervene in middle-aged adults. The beneficial effects of micronutrients (eg vitamins) may be more appropriate for an adult population; it has been suggested that further epidemiological data addressing the role of micronutrients (as well as possible protective effects of fruits and vegetables) in various adult age groups would be helpful. In addition to choosing an age group for which the intervention can be effective, age is also relevant to the feasibility of the study: how many subjects are required and how long must they be followed in order to observe an adequate number of endpoint events? Expressed another way, the sample size and duration depend on the risk of events, and the risk depends on age at randomization.

The risk depends on other factors as well, of course, and prevention trials are often planned to admit only high-risk subjects. There is a trade-off: having stricter criteria (higher risk) for eligibility allows a lower sample size, but may involve more effort and cost in identifying such individuals (in fact, may even involve screening a greater total number of individuals initially, although the number entered is lower).

In gastric cancer, I believe the balance favors choosing a suitably high-risk population. This brings us to consideration of current concepts of gastric carcinogenesis. For the intestinal type, there appears to be a series of entities with an increasing risk of cancer: chronic atrophic gastritis, intestinal metaplasia, dysplasia. More detailed categories can be established based on markers or phenotypic indicators of the precancerous process. The decision of exactly what constitutes the target population is a very important one and must be made with care. The point in the process at which we intervene not only determines what is the expected risk of cancer in such individuals but also affects the possible success of the intervention.

### Specifying the Endpoint

Three types of endpoints have been suggested for gastric cancer prevention studies. In the first situation, individuals with a specified high-risk condition, pre-malignant lesion, or abnormal marker are admitted, and the intervention is administered with the purpose of reversing the condition. I have two comments here. First, it must be realistic to expect that the condition can be reversed in subjects of this age. For example, scepticism exists about proposals to reverse chronic atrophic gastritis in adults. Second, even if the lesion is theoretically reversible, an intervention that has no ability to produce such improvement but does arrest the progression toward higher-risk lesions or more importantly toward malignancy itself is more relevant to our principal goal, and we would not want to fail to identify this.

The second design addresses specifically the progression to higher-risk lesions. For example, one interesting idea is to start with chronic atrophic gastritis and intestinal metaplasia, and attempt to prevent or decrease development of dysplasia (or related markers of pre-malignancy). This type of trial might well yield evidence suggestive of an intervention's capability as a cancer preventive agent.

In the field of cancer treatment trials, it is customary to define Phase II trials as studies to screen new agents for "activity" against tumors; the successful drugs are then candidates for larger Phase III trials which compare therapies for efficacy, often with survival as the definitive endpoint. Although this terminology is not commonly applied to prevention studies, I think it has a useful counterpart in prevention, with the types of trials addressed above being "Phase II" trials to screen for possible "activity".

The two designs described above use endpoints that are surrogates for cancer incidence. Surrogate endpoints are often advocated because they allow studies to be done with fewer subjects and over shorter periods of time. They have increased justification to the extent that cancers develop in a clear progression through the spectrum of high-risk and pre-malignant conditions. Although all cancers may not develop in this way, decrease in occurrence of a surrogate endpoint that represents a condition of increased risk of cancer may still represent a worthwhile contribution to decreasd cancer incidence.

The third type of design is based on cancer incidence as the endpoint. This may be chosen because of questions that arise using surrogate endpoints. First, to what extent might an intervention decrease (or mask) a presumed marker of dysplasia or pre-neoplasia that, in fact, is not directly relevant to development of invasive cancer (although it may be seen more commonly in assocaition with increased cancer risk)? This could lead to a false positive "Phase II" study, thus showing the importance of subsequently confirming positive results in a study with cancer incidence as the endpoint. More worrisome, to what extent might an intervention allow markers of dysplasia to progress as before, but still be effective in preventing the actual development of invasive cancer? This could lead to a false negative "Phase II" study, causing a potentially useful intervention to be discarded. These considerations argue for doing a definitive study with cancer incidence as the endpoint. This requires a large sample size and a longer study, and thus whether it is justified may depend, at least in part, on the strength of our belief that the interventoin is potentially efficacious.

Determining the Sample Size and Trial Duration

The trial must have large enough sample size to ahieve adequate statistical power (probability of having a statistically significant result if in fact the interventions differ in efficacy). For our purposes, the most likely design is a two-arm trial, with one group randomized to receive intervention (consisting of one or multiple components), and the other acting as control. Alternatively, as discussed above, more than one intervention could be studied simultaneously in a factorial design.

The statistical power to detect any specified difference between groups depends on the number of endpoint events expected to occur, and the smaller the difference that we wish to detect, the larger the sample size that is required. To plan the study, or to choose between competing suggestions, there are several pieces of information required. Given the types of subjects specified in the eligibility criteria, what is the expected rate of occurrence of the endpoint? This is a key question needed to determine the number of subjects to be enrolled in the trial and the duration of follow-up. Next, what are the prevalences of the eligibility conditions in the geographic population of interest? This question is relevant to the feasibility of the trial. Finally, what is the difference we expect to find between the randomized intervention arms, and is it realistic to expect that the intervention(s) will produce such a result? This last question is a most important one in any randomized trial, whether therapeutic, diagnostic, or preventive, yet it is often difficult to answer before the trial. Of course, any sample size determination is only an estimate, but unfortunately it is not uncommon for trials to begin with unrealistic estimates and therefore to have unacceptably high probabilities of giving false negative or indeterminate results.

Prevention trials have other considerations, which usually are less of a problem in treatment trials. First, dietary interventions are likely to require a period of time before their benefit will be apparent. This "lag-time" must be considered when designing the trial. Second, compliance in the intervention group may well be less than ideal. This of course can happen in treatment trials also, but probably to a lesser extent than in dietary prevention trials; it may be argued that micronutrient supplementation will lead to better compliance than dietary modifications. Third, it is possible that dietary changes will occur spontaneously in the control group, influenced by other efforts to convince people to improve their health through diet. These various considerations do not necessarily invalidate the trial. The randomized trial still provides an unbiased estimate of how the intervention, as received in practice by the "treated" group, affects the outcome compared to the control ("untreated") group. The important thing is to factor these considerations into the planning of the study, so that the difference that the trial is designed to detect is a realistic one.

CONCLUSIONS

A definitive randomized trial for prevention of gastric cancer would use cancer incidence as an endpoint. This would require a large sample size, but with gastric cancer being a major world problem, in spite of declines over time, such a study may well be possible. The specific definition of eligibility that is agreed upon (eg chronic atrophic gastritis, intestinal metaplasia, evidence of dysplasia) determines the extent of elevated risk and the expected number of cancers. Use of markers such as pepsinogen I (or the ratio of pepsinogen I to pepsinogen II) for atrophic gastritis provides a way to screen the population to determine potential eligibles. Geographically identified high-risk populations could provide sizable numbers of persons with the specified condition(s). In addition, existing epidemiological cohorts or other identified groups, such as the cases (of chronic atrophic gastritis with intestinal metaplasia) in the ECP European collaborative study on the role of diet and other factors in the aetiology of atrophic gastritis, can act as sources of eligible individuals for a randomized intervention trial.

Interventions thought to affect promotion or influence progression from premalignant conditions to cancer could be applied to such persons. Possibilities are addition of fruits and vegetables or administration of certain micronutrients. There may be practical reasons for prefering the micronutrient supplementation over dietary modification. Micronutrients that have been suggested include carotenoids, vitamin C, and vitamin E. More speculative may be an element such as calcium, which has been discussed in terms of colon cancer; does the north/south gradient seen for gastric cancer in some countries have anything to do with vitamin D and calcium? There are other possible explanations, and additional epidemiological studies could address this question.

A decision to be made is whether, before proceeding to a major study with cancer incidence as the endpoint, candidate interventions should be "screened" for activity in a randomized trial with a suitable surrogate endpoint (eg blocking progression in the metaplastic or dysplastic process). Here markers and other phenotypic indicators may play a role, not only in identifying eligibles (eg pepsinogens) but also in defining the endpoint (eg mucins, antigens). Such a trial would also provide valuable information on natural history and rates of progression.

Regardless of which trials are formulated, the challenge here will be in acquiring suitable study populations so that the trials provide adequate tests of the interventions. The use of multicentre and international trials are appropriate ways to obtain large numbers of participants.

REFERENCES
1. Blot WJ, Li J-Y (1985) Natl Cancer Inst Monogr 69:29-34
2. Byar DP, Piantadosi S (1985) Cancer Treat Rep 69:1055-1063
3. Green SB (1981) Semin Oncology 8:417-423
4. Howson CP, Hiyama T, Wynder EL (1986) Epidemiol Rev 8:1-27
5. Parkin DM, Stjernsward J, Muir CS (1984) Bull WHO 62:163-182

© Elsevier Science Publishers B.V. (Biomedical Division)
Gastric carcinogenesis. P.I. Reed, M.J. Hill, editors.

CHEMOPREVENTION

PETER I REED

Gastrointestinal Unit, Wexham Park Hospital, Slough, Berkshire SL2 4HL, UK

INTRODUCTION

Except for the relatively small percentage of cases categorised as early gastric cancer, carcinoma of the stomach carries a poor prognosis and therefore preventive measures are more important than therapeutic ones in mitigating the consequences of exposure to the relative carcinogens. While the past 30-40 years have seen a worldwide reduction in its incidence, gastric cancer is numerically still one of the most important cancers worldwide, generally tending to be seen in lower socio-economic populations, and environmental factors appear to play a most important aetiological role in the intestinal type of gastric cancer.

As the stomach is the first organ to come into prolonged contact with food and drink, and since the human diet contains both carcinogens and anti-carcinogens it is very likely that dietary factors affect the risk of carcinogenesis, and that appropriate modification of the diet might reduce such a risk. Experimental epidemiological studies have suggested a number of possible mechanisms in the pathogenesis of gastric cancer. Of these the most plausible is that proposed by Correa (7) and discussed in detail by him in an earlier chapter (6). The role of vitamins C and E and beta-carotene acting as antioxidants, thereby inhibiting the formation of nitrite from nitrate has already been referred to by Preussmann (26). Another hypothesis concerns tissue stress or damage resulting from the intake of polyunsaturated fat. There is evidence that unsaturated fatty acids participate in peroxidative membrane reactions possibly yielding lipid peroxides which could be involved in carcinogenesis (37). It has also been suggested that consumption of unsaturated fats, particularly linoleic acid, could result during prostaglandin synthesis, in an increase in tissue arachidonic acid, resulting in production of 'active' oxygen radicles which may also particpate in carcinogenesis. Lipid-phase antioxidants such as vitamin E are thought to inhibit both of these processes, probably acting as scavengers of lipid peroxides and 'active' oxygen (19). Similarly, the inhibitory role of marine oils can be explained by their interference with the conversion of linoleic acid into prostaglandins.

In addition to vitamin C, E, beta-carotene and various retinoids, other naturally occuring dietary constituents, a number as yet unidentified, probably act as inhibitors of carcinogenesis. However, for such dietary manipulation to be effective a knowledge of the mechanisms of cancer initiation, promotion, progression and inhibition is a necessary pre-requiste for effective cancer prevention. However, our present state of knowledge of these mechanisms in gastric cancer is still very incomplete.

## ROLE OF MICRONUTRIENTS

For normal cell processes to be maintained essential nutrients of requisite type and in appropriate quantities are required. These are many and diverse and reference has already been made by Diplock (9) to some of these, notably the micronutrients, several of which, including vitamins C, E, A, beta-carotene, retinol and retinyl esters, probably play an important role as natural inhibitors of carcinogenesis. Thus, a consequence of disturbing these processes can be the development of disordered cell behaviour of variable severity, including cancer, which may be associated with abnormal levels of such micronutrients and other substances in the tissues, their serum levels not necessarily being related to relevant tissue concentrations.

Chemoprevention, a relatively new and increasingly important area of cancer research, involves the manipulative use of micronutrients, naturally occuring metabolic products or various appropriate chemicals to reduce cancer incidence. An effective agent might interfere with any of the stages of the neoplastic process involving a variety of mechanisms, such as the inhibition of carcinogen formation from precursor substances, blockage of the effects of carcinogens in critical intracellular sites or suppression of malignant expression after carcinogen exposure. In 1982, following a decade of studying the effects of vitamins on cancer, the US National Cancer Institute (NCI) launched a cancer chemoprevention programme that included support of basic research and clinical trials with vitamins. Concurrently, the American Cancer Society also decided to support chemoprevention research. A very extensive literature has now developed on this subject as over 500 substances have been shown to have some chemopreventive activity, and a number of these are now undergoing in vitro, toxicological and clinical testing. For instance, over 100 animal studies alone confirm the ability of vitamin A and its derivatives to inhibit the development of various cancers (16). Indeed, NCI is currently sponsoring studies of 25 agents (Table 1), mostly chemicals and some vitamins either singly or in combination, chosen primarily on published information of efficacy in preclinical systems for use in chemoprevention of various cancers, including those of the skin, breast, cervix, prostate, colon and oesophagus, and additionally one study looking at all sites (25). Results to date indicate that a number of these compounds look promising for current or eventual clinical evaluation. So far the stomach does not figure in this programme (Kelloff GJ, Personal Communication). However, before any of these agents can be used for chemoprevention in man a knowledge of their toxicology and laboratory evaluation by employing in vitro and in vivo screening utilising a variety of animal models is required.

TABLE 1

CHEMOPREVENTIVE AGENTS (REGIMENS) UNDER STUDY

Beta-Carotene

4-Hydroxyphenyl Retinamide

Selenomethionine

Sodium Selenate

Sodium Selenite

4-Hydroxyphenyl Retinamide + Tamoxifen

4-Hydroxyphenyl Retinamide + Sodium Selenite

4-Hydroxyphenyl Retinamide + Sodium Selenite + Vitamin E

Vitamin E

Sodium Selenite + Vitamin E

Beta-Carotene + Retinol

DHEA Analog(s)

Dehydroepiandrosterone

Proxicam

Bromoergocryptine

Sodium Molybdate

Fluocinolone Acetonide

Difluoromethyl - Ornithine

Hexamethylene Bisacetamide

Dithiolthiones

Ellagic Acid

Benzyl Isothiocyanate

Indole - 3 Carbinol

Butylated Hydroxyanisole

Sulfasalazine

There are difficulties in developing cancer chemoprevention strategies. While it would seem logical to identify high risk populations, to concentrate on these alone may have drawbacks. Again, while many in vitro studies have demonstrated an inhibitory effect on cell transformation of various compounds, including beta-carotene and several retinoids, their application in in vivo animal studies have often proved ineffective in experimentally induced cancer. For instance beta-carotene is ineffective in experimental bladder and tracheal cancer but very effective against breast and lung cancer (24), while selenium is effective only in mammary and oesophageal papillomata (24). Sometimes these compounds may have synergistic effects e.g. in N-methyl-N-nitrosourea (MNU)-induced rat breast cancer, a combination of tamoxifen (an anti-oestrogen) with the retinoid 4-hydroxyphenyl retinamide (4-HPR) is more effective than 4-HPR alone (24).

The effectiveness of a chemoprevention agent will be dependent on various factors, including the timing of its administration following exposure to the carcinogen. For instance, the use of various retinoic acid compounds (RA) was studied in MNU-treated rats, with the RA given at different times after application of the carcinogen over a 26 week period. The results demonstrated a definite time dependency (24). A similar effect was also demonstrated by Santamaria et al (31) in another rat study in which beta-carotene or canthaxanthin was orally administered at different times following the induction of gastric carcinogenesis by low doses of the direct acting carcinogen N-methyl-N-nitro-N'-nitrosoguanidine (MNNG). The results demonstrated that whereas supplemental carotenoids had no influence on initiation or promotion of the pre-neoplastic lesions, they did interfere with progression of the dysplasia to early and infiltrating carcinomas in more than 50% of animals so treated.

However, extrapolation of experimental results to human cancer prevention can be disappointing. Let me cite as an example, Barrett's oseophagus, a premalignant condition in which metaplastic columnar epithelium replaces the normal squamous epithelium of the lower oesophagus. In a recent study (11) the activity of ornithine decarboxylase (ODC), a rate-limiting enzyme in the polyamine biosynthetic pathway and essential for intestinal mucosal proliferation, was demonstrated to have been increased also in dysplastic oesophageal mucosal cells, the cell cultures being obtained from endoscopic biopsies and the effects of various chemopreventive agents tried in vitro. Alpha-difluoromethylornithine proved an effective inhibitor of ODC activity when tested experimentally, but its use in man is unlikely because of dose limiting toxicity, while 13-cis-retinoic acid, generally a very effective antioxidant had no inhibitory effect on cell growth (12). This lack of effect was confirmed in an open short term (6 weeks) clinical study with 13-cis-retinoic acid in a group of 10 patients with Barrett's oesophagus, six of whom had significant complications from this retinoid treatment which had to be discontinued in four as two patients developed oesophageal ulcers and two others mood changes. Halving the dose from 1mg/kg/day was required in two others because of skin toxicity and elevation in serum triglycerides (30). This study also highlighted some of the problems encountered with retinoid treatment, side effects, notably affecting the skin, developing not infrequently.

Another micronutrient employed in intervention studies is beta-carotene, a precursor of vitamin A, which has powerful anti-cancer activity independent of being a pro-vitamin. It acts as an antioxidant, has anti-mutagenic activity, and deactivates potentially carcinogenic free radicals and their precursors. In vitro it has been shown to have an inhibitory effect on cell transformation and also preventing precancerous chromosome damage. A direct effect of beta-carotene supplementation on the reduction of chromosomal aberrations has been demonstrated in regular betel quid chewers in India who are at high risk of developing oral cancer. The administration of beta-carotene alone or together with vitamin A prevented chromosome damage and reduced the number of abnormal buccal mucosal cells by more than 75% (33) and also resulted in a significant remission of oral leukoplakia (34). However, the most dramatic improvement was noted in chewers given regular weekly 200,000 units vitamin A alone for six months in whom no new leukoplastic lesions had developed. Beta-carotene has also been shown to significantly reduce ultraviolet B light-induced skin tumours in animals, especially if pre-treated prior to UV-B exposure (20). This effect is now being applied in intervention studies in Alberta, Canada in patients with previously treated basal cell or squamous cell carcinomas of the skin in whom 25mg beta-carotene daily for two years was unassociated with side effects (32). Another study in Arizona, the state with the highest skin cancer incidence in the USA, employed retinol and 13-cis-retinoic acid as the intervention agents. Concurrently with this, another study was initiated which addressed itself to establishing possible drug-dose responses, an important consideration as drug dosages employed in existing cancer prevention studies generally have not been rationally selected (2).

Other examples of human chemoprevention studies, either completed or in progress, include the use of increasing the dietary calcium intake in high risk groups for colon cancer (35), selenium supplementation in patients in China with primary liver cancer (5), 13-cis-retinoic acid administration in subjects with bronchial atypia (3), and together with alpha-tocopherol in myelodysplasia (4), and trans-retinoic acid in cervical dysplasia (2).

DIET AND GASTRIC CANCER STUDIES

The number of dietary case control (Table 2) and especially chemoprevention studies in gastric cancer is very small. The results of 17 observational studies on diet and gastric cancer have been detailed by Risch et al (29). In general these studies have demonstrated an increased gastric cancer risk with consumption of smoked meats and smoked fish, increased nitrite consumption and lack of refrigeration. These data appear to confirm a role for nitrite in the pathogenesis of gastric cancer. Several studies have documented a protective effect of citrus fruits but in some it is unclear whether this is due to their vitamin C content or some other factor (5). However, a hospital based case-control study in Southern Louisiana of subjects with severe atrophic gastritis in a high risk black population showed a protective effect associated with fruit, vegetables and vitamin C intake, and risk elevation with milk consumption (10). Nevertheless, vitamin C intake calculated from consumption of vegetable does seem to decrease the cancer risk (29), althogh such a relationship has not been demonstrated by others (1,13,15). Beta-carotene has been shown to be weakly protective (29). An increased gastric cancer risk has been observed with consumption of chocolate (23), candy (15) and unsaturated fat consumption, interestingly of oleic rather than linoleic acid (29). In contrast, to the data presented at this symposium by Joossens (18) and Hirayama (17) several studies were unable to support an increased gastric cancer risk with consumption of salt, coffee or alcohol (29). Finally, there have been conflicting reports regarding the effect of dietary fibre intake on the cancer risk (29).

TABLE 2

MODIFIED FROM RISCH ET AL (29)

| Author(s) (Reference No) and year | No of Cases and controls | Country |
| --- | --- | --- |
| Wynder et al 1963 | 521 cases & 653 controls | Japan, New York City Iceland, Slovenia |
| Acheson & Doll 1964 | 100 triples | England |
| Meinsma 1964 | 340 cases & 582+ 478 controls | Netherlands |
| Higginson 1986 | 93 quadruples | United States |
| Graham et al 1972 | 228 pairs | New York State |
| Haenszel et al 1972 | 220 triples | Hawaii |
| Bjelke 1974 | 228 triples 83 triples | Norway Minnesota |
| Modan et al 1974 | 166 cases & 498 controls | Israel |
| Haenszel et al 1976 | 783 pairs | Japan |
| Jedrychowski et al 1980 | 785 pairs | Poland |
| Juhasz 1980 | 338 cases & 553 controls | Eastern Hungary |
| Armijo et al 1981 | 360 pairs | Chile |
| Hoey et al 1981 | 40 cases & 168 controls (all male) | France |
| Ye et al 1981 | 100 pairs | Shanghai |
| Hirayama 1982 | Large cohort | Japan |
| Ikeda et al 1983 | Cohort | Japan |
| Risch et al 1985 | 246 pairs | Canada |

West in his chapter (36) outlined details of an on-going multi-centre, multinational European large scale cohort study comparing the nutritional and micronutrient status of subjects under the age of 55 years with intestinal metaplasia (IM) with matched endoscopic controls without histological abnormalities in the stomach and non-endoscopic controls without gastrointestinal symptoms attending orthopaedic or dermatology clinics. In the four UK centres, various gastric luminal factors as well as plasma levels of several micronutrients, including selenium, vitamins A,C,E and beta-carotene together with pepsinogens and anti-Campylobacter pylori antibody titres are being measured. As yet few data are available, but some interesting information is already forthcoming, notably that a strong geographical North-South gradient in IM incidence is evident.

INTERVENTION STUDIES

To date only three human intervention trials have been carried out. Correa and colleagues (personal communication) recently initiated a pilot feasibility study in a high risk area of Colombia (Narino) studying the possible effect of two months administration of vitamins C, E and A independently on the gastric mucosa in subjects with severe chronic atrophic gastritis. Twenty matched subjects in each of three active treatment groups were compared with a fourth group given placebo tablets. Although no significant histological changes were observed the study did demonstrate good compliance and offers encouragement for carrying out a large scale intervention trial.

In 1983 (27) we reported the results of an intervention study of the effects on the intragastric environment of four weeks treatment with 4g vitamin C daily in 51 hypochlorhydric subjects at high gastric cancer risk due either to pernicious anaemia, chronic atrophic gastritis or following partial gastrectomy. Fasting morning gastric juice samples were obtained before, during and after vitamin C treatment. The mean nitrite ($NO_2$) and total N-nitroso compound (N-NC) concentrations were reduced in the group as a whole, the effect being most marked following partial gastrectomy. Of 55/220 samples found to be mutagenic in the Ames test system 74% were obtained when supplemental vitamin C was not taken. The gastric pH remained virtually unchanged throughout the investigation. A definite deficiency of viatmin C (plasma concentration 2mg/1) was noted in 19/37 patients (51%) in whom vitamin C levels were measured. Subsequently this study was extended to include patients with vagotomy for benign duodenal ulcer and the data re-analysed (28). In four of the five patient groups a definite reduction in $NO_2$ and N-NC concentrations was observed during vitamin C administration but this was not seen in a small group of 9 PA patients, 7 of whom had normal plasma vitamin C levels, in contrast to the 38 surgically treated patients of whom only 30% had normal vitamin C levels. Somewhat unexpectedly vitamin C administration induced a significant reduction in median gastric juice pH during treatment, from 4.5 to 2.4, in both the vagotomy groups (highly selective and vagotomy with drainage), resulting in concurrent inhibition of growth of intragastric nitrate reducing microorganisms. A consequence of this was also the limiting of bacterial reduction of nitrate in the stomach and thereby in the formation of N-NC. As vitamin C undergoes rapid oxidation in the presence of achlorhydria, it could be that vitamin C supplementation of achlorhydric subjects might be unsuccessful in maintaining high gastric ascorbic acid concentrations and could explain the finding in the pernicious anaemia patients in whom the highest gastric pH levels were formed (Schorah CJ pesonal communication). Clearly the number of patients studied was too small for definite conclusions to be drawn and further studies are now in progress to validate these results.

Somewhat similar results were obtained by Kyrtopoulos (21) who supplemented the diet of subjects with 400mg daily each of vitamin C and alpha-tocopherol. This resulted in a significant reduction of mutagenic compounds excreted with faeces suggesting that antioxidants in the diet may have a role in lowering the body's exposure to endogenously formed mutagens.

CONCLUSIONS

Although the data from these three intervention studies are rather meagre, sufficient information is now available about the probable mechanism of gastric carcinogenesis to establish that the intestinal type of gastric cancer is suitable for chemoprevention, and that initiating larger scale intervention trials in high risk cancer populations probably is justified. However, not only do these populations have to be identified but intervention trials have to be very carefully designed, as stressed by Green (14). The gastric lesion most amenable to intervention is probably intestinal metaplasia and possibly also mild dysplasia which at this stage is potentially reversible. The numbers of subjects requiring treatment will have to be sufficiently large to satisfy appropriate statistical criteria. The combination of vitamin C and beta-carotene is probably the most likely way to achieve an histological response.

Finally, the topics which require consideration in identifying new, or re-defining existing directions for chemoprevention as defined by Meyskens (22) are as follows:

1. Definition of the genotypic contribution of the host to cancer risk.
2. Increased understanding of the natural history of human cancer and the attendant phenotypic stresses which promote the process of carcinogenesis or cause pre-neoplasias to progress.
3. Increased biological, biochemical and pharmacological understanding of how

micronutrients and pharmacological agents work.

4. Development of intermediate inpoints or proxies for cancer risk or development.

5. Better laboratory or epidemiological understanding of the interaction of multiple micronutrients as preventive agents.

6. Unified dietary approach to cancer prevention.

In planning future studies additional requirements include:

1. Logical approach to use of chemoprevention agents for cancer prevention trials.

2. the use of multiple micronutrients in one arm of a trial should be continued.

3. Testing of the unified dietary approach to cancer prevention should be undertaken.

4. Further research is required on the design, analysis and interpretation of prevention trials.

It is hoped that the next symposium on gastric carcinogenesis will have a lot more data to offer on these various topics.

ACKNOWLEDGEMENTS

I wish to thank Drs Pelayo Correa and Michael J Hill for many helpful discussions and Mrs Joyce Abraham for typing the manuscript.

REFERENCES

1. Acheson ED, Doll R (1964) Gut 5:126-131

2. Alberts DS, Peng YM, Plezia P, Sayers S, Xu MJ, Davis TP (1988) Third International Conference on the Prevention of Human Cancer: Chemoprevention. Tucson AZ. Abstract S2-3

3. Arnold A, Johnston B, Stoskopf B, Skingley P, Browman G 91988) Third International Conference on the Prevention of Human Cancer: Chemoprevention. Tucson AZ. Abstract S4-6

4. Besa EC, Abraham JL, Nowell PC (1988) Third International Conference on the Prevention of Human Cancer. Chemoprevention. Tucson AZ. abstract S4-13 the Prevention of Human Cancer. Chemoprevention. Tucson AZ. Abstract S4-13

5. Clark LC, Li WG, Yu SY, Zhu YJ, Huang QS (1988). Third International Conference on the Prevention of Human Cancer. Chemoprevention. Tucson AZ. Abstract S3-7

6. Correa P (1988) In: Reed PI, Hill MJ (eds) Gastric Carcinogenesis. Elsevier, Amsterdam pp

7. Correa P, Haenszel W, Cuello C, Tannenbaum S, Archer M (1975) Lancet ii:58-60

8. Dion PW, Bright - See EB, Smith CC, Bruce WR (1982) Mutat Res 102:27-37

9. Diplock AT (1988) In: Reed PI, Hill MJ (eds) Gastric Carcinogenesis. Elsevier, Amsterdam, pp

10. Fontham E, Zavala D, Correa P, Rodrigues E, Hunter F, Haenszel W,

262

Tannenbaum SR (1986) JNCI 76:621-627

11. Garewal H, Prabhala R, Sampliner R, Sloan D (1988) Third International Conference on the Prevention of Human Cancer. Chemoprevention, Tucson AZ. Abstract S1-5A

12. Garewal H, Gerner E, Sampliner R, Alberts D, Roe D (1988) Third International Conference on the Prevention of Human Cancer. Chemoprevention, Tucson AZ. Abstract S1-5B

13. Graham S, Schotz W, Martino P (1972) Cancer 30:927-938

14. Green SB (1988) In: Reed PI, Hill MJ (eds) Gastric Carcinogenesis. Elsevier, Amsterdam pp

15. Haenszel W, Kurihara M, Segi M, Lee RKC (1972) J Natl Cancer Inst 49:969-988

16. Hill DL, Grubbs CJ (1982) Anticancer Res 2:111-114

17. Hirayama T (1988) In: Reed PI, Hill MJ (eds) Gastric Carcinogenesis. Elsevier, Amsterdam pp

18. Joossens JV (1988) In: Reed PI, Hill MJ (eds) Gastric Carcinogenesis. Elsevier, Amsterdam pp

19. King MM, McCay PB (1983) Cancer Res (Suppl) 43:2485s-2490s

20. Krinsky NI (1988) Third International Conference on the Prevention of Human Cancer: Chemoprevention. tucson AZ. Abstract S2-2

21. Kyrtopoulos S (1984) In: Environmental Carcinogens. The problem in Greece. Proc Panhellenic Congress of Greek Society of Preventive Medicine, March 1984

22. Meyskens FL Jr (1988) Third International Conference on the Prevention of Human Cancer. Chemoprevention. Tucson AZ. Abstract S4-15

23. Modan B, Lubin F, Boxall V, Greenberg RA, Modan M, Graham S (1974) Cancer 34:2087-2092

24. Moon RC (1988) Third International Confernce on the Prevention of Human Cancer. Chemoprevention. Tucson AZ. Abstract S1-4

25. Nixon DW (1988) Third International Conference on the Prevention of Human Cancer. Chemoprevention. Tucson AZ. Abstract S1-1

26. Preussmann R, Tricker AR (1988) In: Reed PI, Hill MJ (eds) Gastric Carcinogenesis. Elsevier, Amsterdam pp

27. Reed PI, Summers K, Smith PLR, Walters CL, Bartholopmew B, Hill MJ, Vennitt S, Hornig D, Bonjour J-P (1983) Gut 24:492-493

28. Reed PI, Johnston BJ, Haines K, Walters CL, Hill MJ (1988) Cancer Letters 39 (Suppl March):S34

29. Risch HA, Jain M, Choi NW, Fodor JG, Pfeiffer CJ, Howe GR, Harrison LW, Graib KJP, Miller AB (1985) Am J Epidemiol 122:947-959

30. Sampliner RE, Garewal HS, Meyskens F (1988) Third International Conference on the Prevention of Human Cancer. Chemoprevention. Tucson AZ. Abstract S4-11

31. Santamaria L, Bianchi A, Ravetto C, Arnaboldi A, Santagati G, Andreoni L (1987) J Nutr Growth Cancer 4:175-181

32. Siu TO, Thompson JN, Endo R, Kan S, Nuygen S, Heise M (1988) Third International Conference on the Prevention of Human Cancer, Chemoprevention. Tucson AZ. Abstract S2-4A

33. Stitch HF, Rosin MP (1984) Lancet i:1204-1206

34. Stitch HF, Rosin MP, Hornby AP, Mathew B, Sankeranarayanan R, Krishnan Nair M (1988) Third International Conference on the Prevention of Human Cancer. Chemoprevention. Tucson AZ. Abstract S4-10

35. Wagovich MJ, Faintuch JS, Levin B (1988) Third International Conference on the Prevention of Human Cancer. Chemoprevention. Tucson AZ. Abstract S3-4

36. West CE (1988) In: Reed PI, Hill MJ (eds) Gastric Carcinogenesis. Elsevier, Amsterdam pp

37. Witting LA (1975) Am J Clin Nutr 27:952-959

© *Elsevier Science Publishers B.V. (Biomedical Division)*
*Gastric carcinogenesis. P.I. Reed, M.J. Hill, editors.*

# OVERVIEW

P CORREA

Department of Pathology, Louisiana State University, Perdido Street, New Orleans
LA 70112, USA

Several mesaages appear to surface as we recollect the presentations, discussions and posters of this international symposium. Some are recognitions of facts that are still with us as we appraoch the final years of this 20th century. Others represent the settling of controversies which now seem to reflect more semantic entanglements than biological facts. Still others remind us of important technological improvements and of new scientific discoveries of relevance to the gastric precancerous process.

Hard realities still with us are the following:

In spite of decreasing incidence rate, the latest available statistics show that gastric cancer is still the most frequent malignant neoplasm in the world (skin cancer excluded). Pockets of high risk sub-populations are found in all continents. Prognosis is dismal, except for the "early" cancers which are relatively frequently discovered in Japan but not in most Western societies. These facts reiterate the need for prevention, which requires better understanding of the precancerous process.

Semantic difficulties appear at the center of apparent controversies. One of these is the morphologic and histochemical nomenclature of precancerous lesions. Pathologists with special interest in the subject unanimously recognize the heterogeneity of the metaplastic process and the importance of the more advanced stages in which the presence of sulphomucins deserve attention as a possible preneoplastic marker.

Seemingly, the role of nitrate in the environment seems to be finding its proper place. Clearly it is not the rate-limiting factor of gastric cancer incidence in countries such as England but, equally clearly, it may be an important source of highly reactive gastric nitrite in subjects with chronic atrophic gastritis. The public health aspects of the problem need not interfere with the study of in vivo nitrosation as a potentially pertinent model fo carcinogenesis in humans.

Technological improvements in the detection and identification of N-nitroso compounds have brought much needed light to the search for the relevant chemical compounds (if any) and their precursors. N-nitroso indoles appear as possible common links in populations of great dietary diversity.

Endoscopic technology is being applied to rather large numbers of subjects and contributing to etiologic research in human populations.

New findings of relevance are the better understanding of the pertinent resident flora and the potential role of <u>Campylobacter</u> infection. The role of oxygen radicals has opened new avenues of research which may provide a glimpse to the possible link between the precancerous process and the poorly understood and perhaps not so anachronic theories of "ageing". An epidemiologic hypothesis for the "modulation" of ageing was first heard at this symposium.

The hypothesis of gastric carcinogenesis proposed in 1975 has accomplished its purpose, namely to be scrutinized intensely by international multidisciplinary scientific teams. In spite of serious challenges and some adjustments, the central theme remains today a viable proposition which may be applicable to diverse populations throughout the world. While performing research related to the hypothesis scientists have made important contributions, such as the understanding of <u>in vivo</u> nitrosation, of markers of differentiation, of dietary factors and their timing in the apparently complex chain of causation. It has become now possible to test segments of the hypothesis and to refine epidemiologic techniques to study the interdependence and the chronologic sequence of the multiple biological phenomena involved.

What we learn studying the biology of the gastric precancerous process may be helpful to face the challenges of the next century, for instance as it refers to genetic-environmental interactions, <u>in vivo</u> synthesis of carcinogens and modulation of carcinogenesis in organs other than the stomach.

# INDEX OF AUTHORS